Mind the Science

Mind the Science

Saving Your Mental Health from the Wellness Industry

JONATHAN N. STEA, PhD

OXFORD
UNIVERSITY PRESS

OXFORD
UNIVERSITY PRESS

Oxford University Press is a department of the University of Oxford. It furthers the University's objective of excellence in research, scholarship, and education by publishing worldwide. Oxford is a registered trade mark of Oxford University Press in the UK and certain other countries.

Published in the United States of America by Oxford University Press
198 Madison Avenue, New York, NY 10016, United States of America.

Library of Congress Cataloging-in-Publication Data
Names: Stea, Jonathan N., author.
Title: Mind the science : saving your mental health from the wellness industry / Jonathan N. Stea.
Description: New York, NY : Oxford University Press, [2024] |
Includes bibliographical references and index.
Identifiers: LCCN 2024013883 (print) | LCCN 2024013884 (ebook) |
ISBN 9780197748817 (hardback) | ISBN 9780197748831 (epub) |
ISBN 9780197748848
Subjects: LCSH: Mental health promotion—Social aspects. | Alternative medicine—Social aspects | Pseudoscience. | Mental health. | Well-being.
Classification: LCC RA790.53 .S74 2024 (print) | LCC RA790.53 (ebook) |
DDC 362.2—dc23/eng/20240523
LC record available at https://lccn.loc.gov/2024013883
LC ebook record available at https://lccn.loc.gov/2024013884

DOI: 10.1093/oso/9780197748817.001.0001

Printed by Sheridan Books, Inc., United States of America

To Leslie, Heidi, and Lou—three people I don't mind.

Contents

Author's Note

You'll notice that I reference my former patients to illustrate concepts in some parts of this book. To protect privacy for all, I've modified their demographic data and disguised their names, as well as the names and details of everyone involved in their stories. In a couple of instances, I've cautiously created composites.

It's also important to know that *Mind the Science* has a section at the end of the book called "Mind the Takeaways." It includes material meant to complement the ideas in the main text, but in a format other than prose.

Introduction

The Road to Hell Is Paved With Pseudoscience

Your mental health is precious. You need it to experience joy. You need it to live with purpose, to function in society, and to be there for your loved ones. There's no price tag high enough to measure its value.

It's also fleeting. It ebbs and flows alongside the major events in our lives. We sense it wax and wane as we enter and leave treasured relationships, as we witness the births and deaths of those near us, as we achieve our goals and weather our failures, and as we continue to breathe, slowly in and slowly out, at the mercy of personal tragedies, social injustices, and ungodly disasters.

It's intangible too. It's hard to put our finger on exactly when we're mentally healthy. Mental illness is far less subtle. We feel its gravity on our chests and the hole in our stomachs when depression steals our light. We watch ourselves recoil from life when under the suffocating thumb of omnipresent anxiety. We hear its voice in our heads whispering words of paranoia from the disquieting lips of psychosis. Mental illness is serious. Its management and your mental health are as priceless and complicated as you are.

Yet, your mental health is for sale. You've been told you lack it and it's available for purchase. You just need to buy the latest book with the latest 30-day diet plan, swallow 15 supplements "they" don't want you to know about, cleanse the toxins from your body by following "10 easy steps," spiritually awaken on a 5-day wellness retreat, or undergo the revolutionary new therapy that most doctors haven't heard about. That cheapened, commodified version of mental health is a wolf in sheep's clothing. It's sexy. It's alluring. And it's a sham. It will take you down a yellow brick road paved with pseudoscience, leaving your mental health for dead.

People are vying to toy with and exploit your mental health every day. Many of them aren't aware of their participation. Like marionettes, their strings are pulled by pseudoscientific ideas that transcend their awareness, despite their good intentions—ideas that have become baked into our culture, health care systems, and institutions. For others, your mental health signifies a money grab.

Misinformation is a term referring to claims that aren't deliberately designed to deceive but are nonetheless false, whereas *disinformation*—otherwise known as propaganda—refers to lies. Both are dangerous when applied to mental health, and I've been railing against both for years. The Italian software engineer Alberto Brandolini playfully articulated how I feel. He birthed the internet adage known as Brandolini's law: "The amount of energy needed to refute bullshit is an order of magnitude bigger than that needed to produce it."

Up until now, I've been expending my energy in a scattered way. My day job as a clinical psychologist at a local hospital is to help people who experience severe addiction and mental disorders. But on the side, I've been exposing and debunking pseudoscientific ideas in the mental health space by writing in scientific publications, magazines, and blogs. I've been doing interviews for news stories and podcasts. I've been living and breathing this topic on social media for years, which has allowed me to build a large and engaged platform in the science communication community. On X (formerly Twitter), I'm constantly fielding these kinds of burning questions from the public: "Dr. Stea, is this therapy considered pseudoscience? Is this guy a quack? Is this website a scam? Is this article legitimate?" I decided it was time to compile all the information you need to answer these questions for yourself in one place: this book.

I embarked on this mission because I've seen so many people hurt by pseudoscience. I wanted to create a resource that could be understood and used by everyone. My aim in *Mind the Science* is to educate and embolden those who wish to make informed decisions about their mental health, and to pull back the curtain on the devastating consequence of allowing pseudoscience promoters to target the vulnerable. In a landscape where mental health concerns are at a fever pitch, I want to provide a salutary beacon of hope to those who have been touched by mental illness, have been misled by false marketing, or are simply curious about the relationship between science and mental health.

While it's the mandate of regulatory bodies of various health professions to protect the public from harm, I want you to walk away from this book with a vitally important, perhaps counterintuitive lesson: We cannot rely merely on care providers and regulatory bodies to protect our mental health. The onus is also on us to empower ourselves with knowledge, such that we can protect ourselves from mental health scams, charlatanry, and poor or misguided health practices.

The first section of the book focuses on equipping you with the necessary background. You'll learn about the nature, evolution, and seduction of pseudoscience, and ultimately how to become science and mental health literate, without years of scientific training or any sort of degree. You'll come to understand how a gigantic chunk of mental health misinformation and propaganda can be traced back through history right up to the present collision of the anti-psychiatry movement and the wellness industry. The second section of the book teaches you how to spot misinformation and propaganda. It will shine a light on various pseudoscientific practices, show you the psychological reasons that leave us so vulnerable to believing misinformation, and help you to develop a keen eye for the tactics and tropes that are used to push propaganda in the wellness and alternative medicine communities. The third section will offer solutions, showing the concepts and science behind various evidence-based ways to improve mental health, and teach you what to look for in a new science-informed light when seeking real professional help. In the end, you'll be better positioned to identify mental health misinformation, to steer clear of misguided and predatory practices, and to understand what mental health really means.

Above all, this book is an invitation to mind the science when it comes to taking care of your mental health. What *is* the science? While some pockets of wellness culture have come to loathe the phrase *the science*—insisting that it represents the interests of corrupt gatekeepers who don't care about your suffering—I wish for us to reclaim the term, as it's properly a shorthand phrase to denote the colossal body of rigorous, ongoing, progressive research conducted by scientists around the clock and across the globe. This book rests on the premise that the scientific method is the best tool we have to guide decisions about our mental health needs. Learning how to pay attention to the science protects us, and we ignore it at our peril.

Unlike rocket science, each of us has experience with the topic of mental health, which makes it easier to believe we can assess claims made without evidence and make claims of our own without expertise. But misinformation is worse than no information—and without science, it prevails.

PART 1
YOU'VE BEEN DECEIVED

1

The Evolution and Seduction of Pseudoscience

In 2018, millions of subscribers to Goop—Gwyneth Paltrow's $250 million natural lifestyle company—were introduced to a new promoted product: the $135 Implant O-Rama, a do-it-yourself coffee enema device. The product's website claimed that coffee enemas "can mean relief from depression, confusion, general nervous tension, many allergy related symptoms, and most importantly, relief from severe pain." The company told its consumers: "Ask not what your colon can do for you, but rather, what you can do for your colon." Coffee enemas were even endorsed on Goop by seemingly respectable physicians: namely, a cardiologist, Alejandro Junger, identified as an "adrenal fatigue expert," and "holistic psychiatrist" Kelly Brogan in her *New York Times* bestseller, *A Mind of Your Own: The Truth About Depression and How Women Can Heal Their Bodies to Reclaim Their Lives.*

What's the problem? Well, it turns out that shooting coffee up your bum will not help with depression or any other health concern. Coffee enemas have a long history in the alternative medicine community despite their lack of credible evidence. They were first introduced as a part of the Gerson Therapy, which was developed by a physician, Max Gerson, in the 1930s for the treatment of degenerative diseases, including cancer. Modern proponents of the therapy still claim that coffee enemas work by helping with liver and intestinal detoxification. The scientific reality is that there is no medical theory or body of research supporting the use of coffee enemas, and in fact they can be quite dangerous and result in burns, inflammation, bacteria in the bloodstream, and even death.

Goop subscribers who purchased Kelly Brogan's book about depression were introduced to even more products, services, and "natural treatments for whole-body wellness" beyond coffee enemas. They were told in Brogan's book that a laundry list of supplements was critical to their health and that "unless you are growing your own organic food in a bubble hermetically sealed from the ravages of the modern industrial world, strategic supplementation is almost always going to help you get better and stay better." They were recommended to doubt whether the scientific construct of depression was even real and were warned about the purported dangers of antidepressant medication, Advil, Lipitor, Prilosec, fluoride, fragrances, genetically modified foods (GMOs), antibiotics, vaccines, and birth control pills. In short, they were sold a cornucopia of misinformation.

There exists little evidence to support the vast majority of Brogan's claims. For example, in the American Psychological Association's official clinical practice guidelines for the treatment of depression—which were developed by health professionals from psychology, psychiatry, and primary care, as well as community members who self-identified as having had depression—it's recommended that depression be treated with evidence-based psychotherapies and antidepressants. After reviewing the science, the guidelines don't recommend anything resembling Brogan's unnecessary and expensive testing and supplementing or dietary plan. And of course, there's no mention of coffee enemas.

* * *

I'm a full-time practicing clinical psychologist, adjunct assistant professor in the Department of Psychology at the University of Calgary, researcher, and science communicator, and during the last several years I've cultivated social media in my quest to call out the questionable practices of grifters, such as those peddled by Goop and Kelly Brogan. A brief definition of grifters: A grifter is a swindler. A charlatan. A fake. A snake oil salesman like Clark Stanley, who sold "snake oil liniment" in the late 19th and early 20th centuries as a cure-all for various health conditions—incidentally, it didn't work, and it didn't even contain actual snake oil. A grifter is a person that preys upon the financial and emotional vulnerabilities and health of people to make a profit. Money aside, their motivations can be manifold. Self-deception is certainly one of them, as many even buy into their own pseudo-profound bullshit (believe it or not, that's actually a science term). At the end of the day, regardless of their intentions—even if they believe they're doing the right thing—grifters worsen health outcomes. They sell fake cures, pseudoscience, and false hope—and that's a real problem for anyone needing assistance with mental health or illness.

* * *

Imagine that you're a patient who is experiencing depressive symptoms and other mental health concerns. You feel tired all the time, unmotivated, anxious, and empty. Your appetite is low. You don't know what's wrong; you just know that you're in psychic pain. You want help. You figure that the first step is to get a diagnosis. Your friend tells you that they stumbled upon a great "integrative medicine" clinic on the internet when searching for a massage therapist. The website says that they have a psychologist and a naturopath and that they believe in a "holistic" approach that treats the whole person and the "root cause" rather than "masking the symptoms." You think that sounds reasonable. So you book an appointment. You meet with the psychologist. They are inviting and friendly and use fancy psychological terms when explaining how they can help you. So you go for it and agree to the assessment. You aren't familiar with the tests, but they say they're using a Myers-Briggs Type Indicator (MBTI) and a Rorschach inkblot. You think you might remember those names from movies you've seen but aren't quite sure. They conduct a 2-hour interview with you and ask you about your upbringing. You then see the naturopath, who also asks you about your childhood, as well as your diet. Together, they diagnose you with "adrenal fatigue." They offer you "energy medicine"—specifically, Reiki—to help "balance your energies." And they sell you some homeopathic remedies to help with your tiredness and low appetite. You don't know it just yet—and they might not know it either—but you've just been conned. Adrenal fatigue is a fake diagnosis. It doesn't exist as a recognized medical condition. And both energy medicine and homeopathy are unequivocally pseudoscience: We would literally have to violate the laws of physics for them to work.

As a clinical psychologist, I have encountered many patients who received pseudoscientific assessments and treatments for their addiction and mental health concerns. The tidal wave of pseudoscientific mental health practices originates both within and outside of the mental health professions. The global health and wellness industry has an estimated value of over $5.6 trillion, which includes legitimate sources of health—such as club memberships and exercise classes—as well as alternative medicine products and services that purport to improve health, based on baseless or exaggerated claims and questionable evidence of safety and effectiveness. In the world of mental health care, scientists have estimated that there are at least 600 "brands" of psychotherapy, an unreasonably and quickly growing number. Beyond that world exist countless unregulated providers of mental health–related services in the wellness industry and alternative medicine community who market themselves as "life coaches," "wellness consultants," and—depending on particular countries and jurisdictions—other various non–legally protected titles, such as "therapists," "psychotherapists," "counselors," and "practitioners."

Snake oil salesmen, then, in the spirit of Clark Stanley, never went away. The debate about what constitutes pseudoscience is as old as science itself. At least as old as Aristotle, the philosophy of science as a discipline of study rose to the fore in the 19th and 20th centuries, as scientists made tremendous advances in fields as diverse as genetics, geology, physics, and health. It was during this time that many individuals, groups, and theories were accused of being pseudoscientific, such as astrology, creationism, and believers in the paranormal.

Historically, the world of mental health has had its own accusations of pseudoscience, notably in the cases of phrenology, an attempt to understand mental life by linking personality traits with skull shape, and

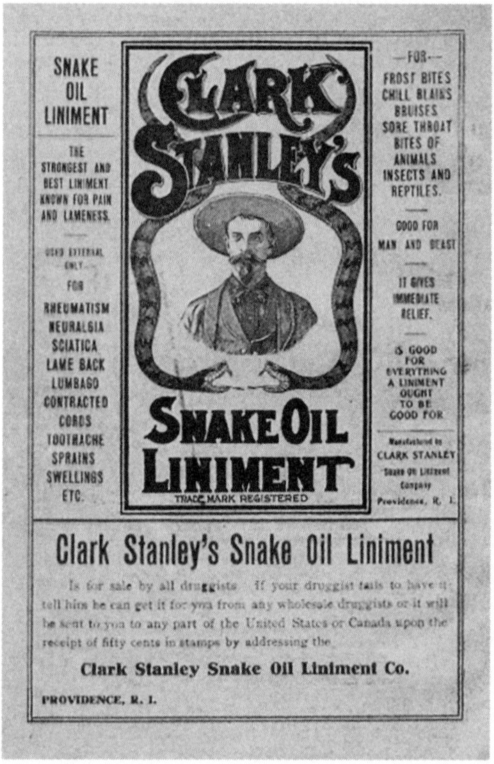

Clark Stanley's Snake Oil Liniment, circa 1905.

Sigmund Freud's psychoanalysis, an attempt to treat mental illness based on Freud's theories of the mind. While phrenology perished in the sands of time, psychoanalysis survived by eventually morphing into a modern evidence-based treatment approach called psychodynamic therapy. In the late 16th and early 17th centuries, Franz Anton Mesmer gained many followers by "mesmerizing" and claiming to heal by aligning magnetic forces, a practice that was a precursor to modern hypnosis. The field of psychiatry fared no better with its claims of treating mental illness with spinning chairs, bloodletting, leeching, prefrontal lobotomies, casket-like Utica cribs, hot and cold baths, purging, blistering, dental removal, mercury dosing, and many other treatments, which are now recognized as useless or harmful.

Pseudoscience is a nebulous term. In short, it is a hijacked and failed attempt at science. But that definition doesn't quite capture its complexity. The first thing to understand about differentiating science from pseudoscience is that there is no single, clear criterion that tells one from the other. Nor is there a single person who can make that call. This problem—of trying to figure out whether a particular discipline, treatment, assessment tool, or research program falls under the purview of pseudoscience—is known in science as the "demarcation problem." In other words, where do we demarcate, or draw the line between, science and pseudoscience? While philosophers of science have been wrestling with the demarcation problem for centuries, I find it useful to understand pseudoscience as best identified by a cluster of warning signs, such that science differs from pseudoscience in degree rather than in kind. I'll introduce you to these warning signs in Chapter 5.

Scott O. Lilienfeld was a modern giant in the field of clinical psychological science and devoted much of his career to elucidating and exposing pseudoscientific practices in the field of psychology. He and his colleagues offered a metaphor for anyone stumped by the demarcation problem. They compared the distinction between science and pseudoscience to the boundary between day and night: The fact that the precise boundary is unclear does not imply that the two cannot be meaningfully differentiated.

No one grows up dreaming of becoming a pseudoscientist, and no one wants to be labeled one either. The truth is that the label itself matters much less than the reasons why something might be considered pseudoscientific. Instances of unequivocal pseudoscience serve as a distorted mirror warning against what not to do scientifically. In other cases, that gray zone in which we're left to decide whether pseudoscience has reared its deceptive head is supposed to be muddy—but it gives us cause to pause, and to proceed with caution when critically thinking about claims related to mental health.

* * *

Fast forward to present day: Mental health pseudoscience and misinformation permeate both popular and social media, as well as our health care systems and its margins. How did we get here? The onset of the Covid-19 pandemic sparked an explosion of health misinformation that the World Health Organization dubbed an "infodemic." And it's no wonder. The American astronomer Carl Sagan predicted in 1995 that pseudoscience and superstition would seem year by year more tempting whenever we experience periods of existential uncertainty. This onslaught of misinformation has extended beyond the issue of Covid-19 to all matters of health, including mental health.

For example, one recent study analyzed popular videos about attention-deficit hyperactivity disorder (ADHD) on the social media platform TikTok, which boasts 1 billion monthly active users. The researchers found that over half of the videos analyzed were misleading, and staggeringly, that there were over 2.8 million views per video and each video was shared on average 31,000 times. Some of the misleading claims in the videos described nonexistent symptoms of ADHD, such as "anxiety shivers," "random noise making," and "being competitive," whereas others inaccurately stated that those who experience ADHD are "only either understimulated or overstimulated" and "lack dopamine."

Countless pseudoscientific practices are now in use for assessing and treating mental illness and improving mental health. While a universally agreed-upon way to categorize them doesn't exist, Chapter 7 is devoted to helping us spot unequivocal instances of pseudoscience and also controversial ones, the latter being more scientifically plausible but still plagued by some pseudoscientific features and low-quality evidence to support their use. A simple Google search of "alternative medicine" and "mental health" unearths many examples from both categories.

Some examples of unequivocal pseudoscientific practices and controversial ones:

Pseudoscientific Practices	Controversial Practices
• Ayurveda	• Animal-assisted therapies
• Biosound therapy	• Cannabis
• Chelation therapy	• Hypnosis
• Chiropractic	• Mindfulness meditation
• Conversion therapy	• Psychedelics
• Energy medicine	• Purple hat therapies
o Cranial-sacral therapy	o Eye movement desensitization and reprocessing (EMDR)
o Emotional freedom techniques	
o Polarity therapy	• 12-step programs, such as Alcoholics Anonymous (AA)
o Reiki	
o Therapeutic touch	
o Thought field therapy	
• Facilitated communication	
• Hyperbaric oxygen therapy	
• Naturopathy	
o Acupuncture	
o Homeopathy	
o Orthomolecular medicine	
• Neurolinguistic programming	
• Ozone therapy	
• Past life regression therapy	
• Scientology's Narconon program	

Rather than trying to thoroughly debunk each example, it can sometimes be more helpful to undermine the theoretical underpinnings of an entire pseudoscientific approach. For instance, people might look to "energy medicine" modalities, such as Reiki, to assist with their mental health concerns. Unfortunately, we'll see why there's no scientific evidence supporting the existence of the energy field thought to play a role in Reiki, nor for other energy medicine practices that claim it exists, such as cranial-sacral therapy, therapeutic touch, polarity therapy, and tapping via emotional freedom techniques and thought field therapy.

Naturopathy is an umbrella term that captures a variety of pseudoscientific practices, such as acupuncture, homeopathy (sometimes referred to as the "air guitar of medicine" because it postulates that a remedy becomes more effective when the active ingredient has been diluted out of existence), and orthomolecular medicine (sometimes referred to as megavitamin therapy). Central to naturopathy is the idea of vitalism, which is scientifically implausible and akin to a magical life-giving energy force that we'll learn about in Chapter 7.

Other times, specific pseudoscientific practices can be called out on their own. On one of my X (formerly Twitter) threads about chiropractic, someone once commented: "In mommy groups on Facebook, they really do think it can cure everything from heartburn to ADHD. I just saw in a breastfeeding group that someone asked for recommendations for a chiropractor who can give her newborn an adjustment to fix their latch." In Chapter 7, I'll tell you why much of chiropractic is pseudoscientific, in addition to other practices. I'll also tell you about the gray zones of cannabis and psychedelic therapy; 12-step programs like Alcoholics Anonymous (AA); animal-assisted therapies; hypnosis and its variants like past life regression therapy; mindfulness meditation; and something called purple hat therapies like eye movement desensitization and reprocessing (EMDR). Ultimately, however, debunking specific pseudoscientific practices can feel like playing the arcade game Whac-A-Mole, where new ones keep sprouting up, which is why it will also be fruitful for us to understand and address the underlying pseudoscientific features, as well as how to evaluate the credibility of scientific evidence; we'll learn about these concepts in Chapters 2, 5, and 6.

But let's take a step back. I'm sometimes asked: What gives? Why are people eating up these pseudoscientific practices in the first place? Why, by one estimate, is the global market for alternative medicine—where many of these practices thrive—projected to be worth nearly $200 billion in 2025? In other words, what makes pseudoscience so tempting? The answer is not simple. There are many potentially related reasons that can interact and account for why so many people find pseudoscience attractive.

A big one is the unfortunate reality that not all legitimate treatments work for everyone. Even some of our best evidence-based treatments, such as cognitive-behavioral therapy (CBT) and antidepressant medication, won't be helpful for many people. It would be absurd to blame someone for seeking alternatives. And as a practicing clinical psychologist who is unable to help all of my patients, I empathize, and I get it.

I've lived it too.

"Jonathan, you just wait until the day that you get sick because then you'll really understand why alternative medicine has its place." On social media, my crusade against pseudoscience has at times been met with sentiments along those lines. They're right. I have been blessed with good health throughout my life. Unfortunately, I can't say the same about my family.

One day when I was 11 years old, I couldn't find my mother anywhere in our house. I finally located her in the bathroom, eyes shut, hunched over while sitting on the toilet with a full cigarette in hand. It had burned out but retained its slightly curved shape as pure ash. A couple of remnants had fallen and left black burns on the tiled floor. This wasn't the first time she'd fallen asleep on the toilet. That tended to happen after I injected her with meperidine (an opioid painkiller) and diazepam (a benzodiazepine sedative).

My mother had been suffering with health problems for years. Nerve damage from a botched spinal surgery had left her with a diagnosis of complex regional pain syndrome: a severe, chronic health condition accompanied by sensory and motor abnormalities and excruciating pain. The condition itself has fascinated scientists and puzzled clinicians for decades due to an incomplete understanding of its complicated nature—so much that even its existence as a distinct diagnostic entity has been questioned in the scientific literature. Academic exercises in diagnosis notwithstanding, I saw the reality of her symptoms with my own eyes, and I was terrified: Her cold, bluish hands, legs, and feet would double in size due to swelling and leaked lymphatic fluid, and she would shriek if water or even wind touched them because it felt like adding gasoline to a body that was already burning. She had other categories of medical symptoms too. For example, I would frequently wake in the middle of the night to her screaming the word "stars!" The yell was a preamble—it meant that violent seizures resembling sit-ups were about to occur.

During my childhood and adolescence, it seemed like she spent more time in the hospital than at home. As an only child growing up in a tight-knit household, my tasks—when my father was at work—were to clean her blistering wounds and help administer her medications so that she could feel some respite. In hindsight, I can't remember how many times I injected her, and neither could she: She became so cognitively impaired by the combination of opioids, benzodiazepines, and pain that we inadvertently doubled and tripled her prescribed doses. She quickly became physiologically dependent on and addicted to her medications. She became depressed, and when I gazed into her eyes I could no longer see my loving mother: She was in there, but she was far away.

My father was at his wits' end. The diagnoses given to my mother were iffy and in flux. Treatment felt hopeless. Mainstream health care was failing us. It seemed like surgeries and medications just added more problems. What would any reasonable people do? We looked to alternatives: acupuncture, herbal remedies, reflexology, chiropractic, detox foot baths, Reiki, therapeutic touch, meditation, past life regression therapy, Rolfing, ear candling, healing crystals, cleansing bells, incense cleanses, psychics, and more.

Alternative medicine didn't help. Some practices—like acupuncture, chiropractic, and detox foot baths—made her feel worse. To this day, we remain at the mercy of the limits of science and a chronic health condition with no known cure. My mother still experiences pain, but she manages it with a variety of approaches, such as anticonvulsant and nonopioid pain medications, activity pacing, relaxation techniques, and exercise. The passage of time has also kindly lifted the roar of her symptoms, which is consistent with the variable prognosis of complex regional pain syndrome, as documented in the scientific literature. She currently enjoys a life free from depression, aided by skills she learned from self-help materials based on CBT and pain management with acceptance and commitment therapy (see Chapter 8).

But it's hard not to feel the stirs of resentment toward mainstream health care. Science can send us to the moon, but my mother was forced into a decades-long trek through a fog of health uncertainty that felt unguided because the offerings of scientific knowledge and effective treatments for what ailed her fell short. I too will get sick one day. Will I reach for the healing crystals? Maybe. Desperation is intoxicating.

The seduction of pseudoscience runs deeper, however, right to the psychological and cultural lens through which we view our world. One U.S. study published in the prestigious *JAMA* (*Journal of the American Medical Association*) suggested that even more important to alternative medicine seekers than being dissatisfied with mainstream health care is finding pseudoscientific practices that are more congruent with their own values, beliefs, and philosophical orientations. If we simply ask people why they use alternative medicine, they'll tell us. They'll say that natural treatments are better than chemical ones—even though such an *appeal to nature* is a known logical fallacy: the false belief that what is natural is good. One could argue that coronaviruses are natural, but they're hardly good. They'll tell us other reasons too: Mainstream health care professionals don't spend enough time with them, they aren't viewed as a whole person, they want to avoid the side effects of medications, the pharmaceutical industry is solely profit driven, among other very justifiable and understandable reasons. And as you'll learn in Chapter 6, we're captivated by fake science news for other psychological and social reasons, such as being victims of our own cognitive biases, the structure of online social networks, and being preyed upon with misinformation and propaganda by grifters and organizations.

What's more, not everyone has access to effective treatment in the first place. Widespread systemic barriers in mainstream health care also play a major role in the triumph of pseudoscience, leading to a lack of easy access to quality care, especially among minority and underprivileged groups. Scientists have estimated that more than 50% of people worldwide who experience mental disorders don't receive treatment at all when they need it—and this estimate approaches a whopping 90% in undeveloped countries. When people are prevented from getting the treatment they need—due to reasons such as lack of insurance coverage, stigma, mental health workforce shortages, unequal distribution of services based on location, and lack of skilled clinicians—pseudoscience peddlers see a green light to slither in and open for business.

* * *

You might ask yourself, "So what? If people think pseudoscientific practices help, then who cares?" Unfortunately, the reality is that pseudoscience is not an innocent game. It's harmful in at least three ways. It can produce harm directly as a result of the therapies used, it can indirectly take hard-earned money and time away from people, and it can further erode the scientific foundations and trust in professions that tolerate its use. Let's unpack those points.

Candace Newmaker was 10 years old when she died on April 19, 2000, covered in her own feces and vomit. Her adoptive mother stood by as two social workers and two assistants wrapped Candace from head to toe in a blue flannel sheet and smothered her with pillows to simulate birth contractions. She was undergoing a 70-minute session of "rebirthing therapy" to treat her reactive attachment disorder. She was airlifted to a local hospital and was pronounced dead of asphyxiation the next morning. The social workers were convicted of reckless child abuse resulting in death and received 16-year prison sentences. Neither of them had an active registration at the time to practice psychotherapy. Candace's adoptive mother, Jeane Newmaker, a nurse practitioner, pleaded guilty to the same charges and was given a 4-year deferred sentence after which the charges were expunged from her criminal record. Following the case, "Candace's Law" was enacted in Colorado and North Carolina, banning all psychotherapies from using active restraint.

Candace shouldn't have died. Reactive attachment disorder is very rare and contentious, as it's seen in less than 10% of cases involving even the most severely neglected children. It's characterized by a pattern of disturbed and developmentally inappropriate attachment behaviors, which essentially means that a child doesn't show consistent effort to obtain comfort, support, nurturance, or protection from their caregivers. The diagnosis and treatment of reactive attachment disorder is complex and needs to be conducted by mental health professionals who are trained and qualified to do so.

Rebirthing therapy is a pseudoscientific treatment invented in the 1970s by Leonard Orr, an alternative medicine guru who pitched the practice predominantly as a breathing technique that is rarely supposed to last more than 15 minutes. The idea is that a child's attachment problems with their caregivers stem from a traumatic birth and that re-enacting this trauma mends previously unprocessed conflicts and emotions. There's no scientific evidence that rebirthing therapy is beneficial for childhood behavioral problems. The therapy used on Candace was a longer 70-minute variant designed to mimic the birth process by regressing her to the moment of her birth and instructing her to fight her way out of the womb while repeatedly squeezing her to relive the trauma. It was part of a $7,000 two-week package, which ultimately involved taunting and crushing her with a combined weight of 304 kg. To my dismay, rebirthing therapy training workshops are still plentily available today.

A similarly tragic case of direct harm involved the death of Kellie Poole, a 39-year-old mother of three children, on April 25, 2022, following a session of "cold water therapy." At the direction of Kevin O'Neill, a non–mental health professional who regularly offers cold water therapy to celebrities, Kellie submerged herself in freezing cold water and then collapsed and died. Cold water therapy is currently advertised on Kevin's website and at the time of writing this book in 2023 was promoted as being able to "help severe PTSD or anxiety sufferers step away from prescribed medications." While some people might recreationally enjoy a cold-lake dip before hitting a sauna, research indicates that cold water therapy can be dangerous, as it can induce a high incidence of cardiac arrhythmias. And there's absolutely no credible evidence to suggest that it's a recommended treatment for posttraumatic stress disorder (PTSD) or anxiety disorders. My heart extends not only to Kellie and her family but also to Kevin, who expressed publicly his devastation over the death. Pseudoscience creates countless victims.

Granted, not all pseudoscientific therapies directly result in death. More often, they can do more subtle harm, such as worsening mental health or illness.

One strong example is the use of "critical incident stress debriefing (CISD)," sometimes referred to as "psychological first aid," which is a pseudoscientific therapy that has been widely promoted to help people—including emergency responders—after they've been exposed to or involved in a potentially traumatic event, such as a fire or car accident. The intention behind CISD is noble: It's designed to prevent the development of PTSD and anxiety disorders after experiencing a traumatic event by encouraging people to discuss and process their thoughts and feelings. The debriefing usually occurs in small groups led by facilitators within 24 to 72 hours after the traumatic event, typically either as a single session lasting 3 to 4 hours or spread out over several sessions. While this therapy has been promoted on popular podcasts, such as *The Joe Rogan Experience*, and continues to be used to this day, strong scientific evidence shows that it can actually worsen posttraumatic stress and anxiety symptoms, perhaps by interfering with the flow of recovery processes that typically occur with the passage of time. Many CISD proponents exhibit two pseudoscientific warning signs: They say that every single person exposed to such a traumatic event can benefit from the intervention, and they dismiss the research showing harm, blaming it on poor clinician training or failure to apply the intervention properly. In Chapter 5, we'll learn that these warning signs correspond to "no stated limitations to the treatment" and "overuse of ad hoc hypotheses," respectively.

Not all harm derived from pseudoscientific therapies is direct. The cost to your well-being could be both financial and intangible. That is, people can dump a wealth of cash and time into pseudoscientific therapies, and while they're watching their wallets dwindle, their mental health or illness symptoms could be getting worse. Rather than suffering, they could've been seeking evidence-based care.

Examples abound of pseudoscience misdirecting those who need real mental health care. For instance, it's not uncommon to hear about the use of over-the-counter supplements or "natural remedies" for the treatment of obsessive-compulsive disorder (OCD). But the best, evidence-based treatment we have for OCD is a CBT approach called exposure and response prevention, which involves helping patients to systematically and safely expose themselves to situations that induce obsessions while not engaging in compulsions. Similarly, a potentially deadly application of an unsupported therapy for opioid addiction is the use of nutrient-based therapies—such as vitamin C—if these therapies are used instead of evidence-based treatments, namely opioid agonist therapies. The very last thing that we want to do is to mismanage opioid addiction in the midst of an overdose crisis in North America. The list goes on: First-line evidence-based treatment for schizophrenia involves antipsychotic medication, not solely diet management or an unsupported type of psychotherapy; it's stimulant medication for ADHD, not chiropractic care; it's CBT for depressive disorders, not Reiki; and it's prolonged exposure and cognitive processing therapy for PTSD, not past life regression therapy—all first-line treatments of which we'll visit in Chapter 8.

The problem lies not simply with the use of pseudoscientific therapies. It's that many of them are given life by pseudoscientific ideas that are entrenched in the wellness industry. We'll see throughout this book how alternative medicine isn't just a mishmash of unsupported and pseudoscientific approaches, but an organized and identifiable ideology. It's a body of longstanding recurring ideas about health that continue to ooze through our culture and that are commercialized and sold to us as wellness. These ideas often portray alternative medicine as a substitute for, equal to, or better than mainstream medicine.

You've likely met people who speak the language of this ideology. They will talk about the horrors of "Big Pharma"—a term referring to the trillion-dollar pharmaceutical industry—and may be convinced that natural and holistic approaches to health are safer and superior to the surgical butchering and pill-popping approach of mainstream medicine. My own patients have been targeted with this kind of messaging.

One of them was immersed in the alternative medicine community on social media. She also happened to experience severe, all-consuming anxiety. If you were able to peek into her world, you would see her surfing websites such as WebMD over 10 times per day to check whether physical symptoms like an upset stomach meant she had diseases like cancer. After reading Facebook posts about other people's health conditions, she would restlessly pace around her apartment, biting her nails, fraught with worry that she too may be afflicted. Relationships with the people in her life became strained as her conversations revolved solely around her health status. We did our due diligence: I encouraged her to connect with her family physician and medical specialists to rule out any physical ailments she may in fact have, but the reassurance she consistently received wasn't enough to pacify her preoccupation with the disease that was the flavor of the week. She told me she felt like a miserable shell of who she used to be. Diagnostically, she was experiencing a type of hypochondriasis that's now called illness anxiety disorder.

Heightening and playing into her anxiety were ideas she believed about her health—ideas that were backed by her online community and legitimized by her naturopath. For instance, she was convinced that if she could just avoid and detox from the toxins in her environment, then she could achieve optimum health. This led her to purchase multiple detox products promising to cleanse and heal. When I decided to Google one of them called Pure Body Extra, even *I* became anxious.

It's a mouth spray containing a liquid form of the dietary supplement *zeolite Clinoptilolite*. Touted as an "all-natural full-body detox" with "advanced nanotechnology" ensuring "benefit with just 4 taste-free sprays, 3 times a day," an advertisement for it reads:

> Exposure to toxins starts even before we're born. From the womb onwards we're surrounded by chemicals, over 80,000 by most counts. This toxic overload continues throughout our lives with toxins in food, water, and even the air we breathe. Pure Body Extra to the rescue. . . . Numerous studies attest to the selective nature of the zeolite Clinoptilolite, to ONLY take out toxins, and never any good nutrients. Our proprietary cleansing process loads the zeolite with beneficial minerals so it always replaces a bad toxin with a good mineral for optimal well-being.

That marketing ploy is clever. It's designed to induce fear and anxiety and then offer a solution. But is there any truth to it? To find out, I spoke to toxicologist and emergency medicine physician Ryan Marino. Who better to ask than someone who specializes in toxic poisonings? He told me:

> Almost any time someone mentions the word *toxins*, you can assume they're not being factual. Everything can be toxic, including oxygen, water, sodium, glucose, and many other things essential to life. Thankfully, even scary-sounding things that can be toxic—like arsenic, formaldehyde, and even heavy metals—are also usually nontoxic in the small amounts in which they're encountered in our diets and everyday life. The rare exceptions prove

> the rule that there's really no such thing as *detoxing*. Your liver and kidneys are the best detox agents you have, and if those aren't working, then you should seek medical attention. While zeolites are unlikely to cause harm if ingested, there's no evidence, or even a theoretical mechanism, to suggest they can treat any medical condition, with one single exception: use for hemorrhage control, since their ability to absorb water from blood allows concentration of clotting factors—and even this is usually reserved for extreme injuries and extreme situations, like austere combat environments.

Marino's insights are damning to every detox product sold in the wellness industry and are consistent with research suggesting that there's no compelling science supporting the use of detox diets for eliminating "toxins" from the body. Pseudoscientific ideas about health can't be blamed as the only cause of my patient's illness anxiety disorder, but they certainly made it worse, and challenging them became a focus of our psychotherapy sessions to help manage her anxiety.

Finally, at its most abstract level, pseudoscience is harmful to society. A culture that tolerates and elevates pseudoscience will be at odds with the health of its citizens. There's perhaps no better example of how pseudoscience has made us sick than observing how it's been wielded by wellness gurus within the anti-vaccine movement in their attempt to undermine efforts to end the Covid-19 pandemic, a topic we'll consider in Chapters 2 and 4. When mental health professions allow pseudoscience to thrive, it erodes their scientific foundations and results in mistrust toward its practitioners. Time, money, and effort are better invested in evidence-based training programs and care. And given that mental health professions, such as clinical psychology and psychiatry, are philosophically, rightfully, and ethically scientific disciplines, it's paramount that both individual practitioners and their regulatory bodies respect and step up to that fact in order to minimize harm.

Pseudoscience is as old as science, and it will continue to be with us because there are many attractive psychological, social, cultural, and economic forces at work in its service. But that doesn't mean that pseudoscience is clinically effective or that it should be tolerated. The deceptions of mental health–related pseudoscience in particular have avoided widespread public exposure and critique—until now.

Carol Tavris, a prominent social psychologist and bestselling author, once paraphrased Richard McNally, a Harvard-based clinical psychologist, as being fond of saying, "The best way to combat pseudoscience is to do good science." Others, including Scott O. Lilienfeld, have argued that it's more than that: It's also knowing how to spot pseudoscience and the ways in which claims are wielded. The best way to protect your mental health is to understand what both good science and pseudoscience look like so that you know which treatments and services to seek and which to avoid. What's the first step? It's becoming literate in both science and mental health, which is exactly what I'll help you do in the next chapter. Armed with an understanding of science and mental health literacy, you will be better prepared to respond to your loved ones if they ask you whether they should buy Kelly Brogan's book or spend $135 on the Implant O-Rama, both of which are still available on Goop's website.

2

Becoming Literate in Science and Mental Health

On December 15, 2005, American comedian, actor, political commentator, and television host Bill Maher appeared on CNN's *Larry King Live*, which at that time was a television show that boasted millions of viewers on a nightly basis. In the middle of the episode, the host, Larry King, asks Bill Maher, "Worried about the avian flu?" Here's what transpired next:

MAHER: Not the least. You know my theory about health.

KING: What?

MAHER: Well, we've talked about it. I'm not into Western medicine. That to me is a complete scare tactic. It just shows you, you can...

KING: You mean you don't get a...you don't get a flu shot?

MAHER: A flu shot is the worst thing you can do.

KING: Why?

MAHER: Because it's got...it's got mercury.

KING: It prevents flu.

MAHER: It doesn't prevent. First of all, that's...

KING: I haven't had the flu in 25 years since I've been taking a flu shot.

MAHER: Well, I hate to tell you, Larry, but if you have a flu shot for more than 5 years in a row, there's 10 times the likelihood that you'll get Alzheimer's disease. I would stop getting your...

KING: What did you say?

MAHER: That went better in rehearsal but it was still good. Absolutely, no, the defense against disease is to have a strong immune system. A flu shot just compromises your immune system.

KING: So you don't take any Western medicine, don't take an aspirin?

MAHER: Never, an aspirin no. Thousands of people die from aspirin every year.

KING: How do you treat illness?

MAHER: I promise you that if you get a headache the reason for that headache is not aspirin deficiency. The reason...

KING: No, of course not.

MAHER: Right, so you're taking... so it's not...

KING: Something to take the pain away. Why is that bad?

MAHER: But why don't you find out the real root of that pain?

KING: Well, while you're finding take the aspirin.

MAHER: But that's what we do. We have immediate cures that address the symptom and not the root cause of anything. I have no worries about bird flu whatsoever. First of all, it's not going to happen. Second of all, the fact that it is mutating shows that if you did come up with a vaccine tomorrow, it wouldn't be effective against the disease when the disease comes because the disease is always morphing and mutating. It's just a way to funnel money into the pharmaceutical companies. Follow the money. You'll find out where the bird flu is.

What's going on here? Is there any merit to Maher's claims? To understand his opinion, we need to take a step back and examine what's informing his views. He provided more clarity about his health beliefs on his hit HBO television series, *Real Time With Bill Maher*, on March 4, 2005, when he stated:

> I don't believe in vaccination either. That's a... well, that's a... what? That's another theory that I think is flawed, and that we go by the Louis Pasteur theory, even though Louis Pasteur renounced it on his own deathbed and said that Béchamp was right: it's not the invading germs, it's the terrain. It's not the mosquitoes, it's the swamp that they are breeding in.

It's here that we see that Maher is actually alluding to a more-than-160-year-old rivalry between two competing theories about how people become sick: Louis Pasteur's "germ theory" versus Antoine Béchamp's "terrain theory." In one corner of the 19th century, we have Pasteur, a French chemist, considered by some to be the father of microbiology. It's hard to find a more decorated contributor to modern medicine and public health, as his research unearthed principles underpinning vaccination and various hygiene practices that prevent disease. His discovery that heating liquids prevents bacterial contamination—known as pasteurization—is also the reason you don't die when you drink milk along with your breakfast cereal or coffee.

In the other corner, we have his contemporary opponent, Béchamp, who was also a French chemist, and who hated Pasteur. If the 19th century had reality TV, science nerds worldwide, including myself, would undoubtedly be entertained when Béchamp stated that Pasteur's views of disease were "the greatest scientific silliness of the age."

So what's the beef? It turns out that Pasteur's and Béchamp's theories were essentially diametrically opposed to one another at the time. Pasteur popularized and scientifically supported germ theory, which is the idea that germs cause disease. In germ theory, "germs" refer to microorganisms such as bacteria and also include viruses—despite the fact that nowadays biologists generally and technically do not consider viruses to be alive, as they exist in the gray zone between organic structures we recognize as being alive and nonliving organic structures. Béchamp's ideas, on the other hand, laid the foundation for terrain theory, which suggests that the body's "terrain," not germs, cause disease. In other words, it's the body of the unhealthy organism that's the disease culprit—microorganisms are a consequence of disease, not its cause.

Two centuries later, the undisputed winner, of course, is germ theory. The stunning success of antibiotics and vaccination is a feather in its cap. Though, modern incarnations of terrain theory complement rather than refute germ theory, as we know, for example, that healthy bodies can better fight the invasion and ravages of germs than unhealthy bodies can.

No credible scientist or health professional today disputes germ theory. And yet, some people do, and their voices can be loud and far reaching. Germ theory denialism is the pseudoscientific belief that germs do not cause disease and that germ theory is wrong. Many public science communicators, such as oncologist David Gorski, have been sounding the alarm bells for decades with respect to the harm associated with germ theory denialism. Since 2008, Gorski, along with neurologist Steven Novella, has managed the popular skeptic website *Science-Based Medicine*, which has shown repeatedly how germ theory denialism thrives in the alternative medicine and anti-vaccine communities.

To get a feel for what it's like being in these communities, you can go directly to the source. For example, on Facebook, I joined the group "Terrain Model Refutes Germ Theory." In Figure 2.1, you can see that as of August 30, 2022, the group had over 26,500 members. And look at a snapshot of the content: The main photographic banner of the group depicts an apple next to a pile of pills,

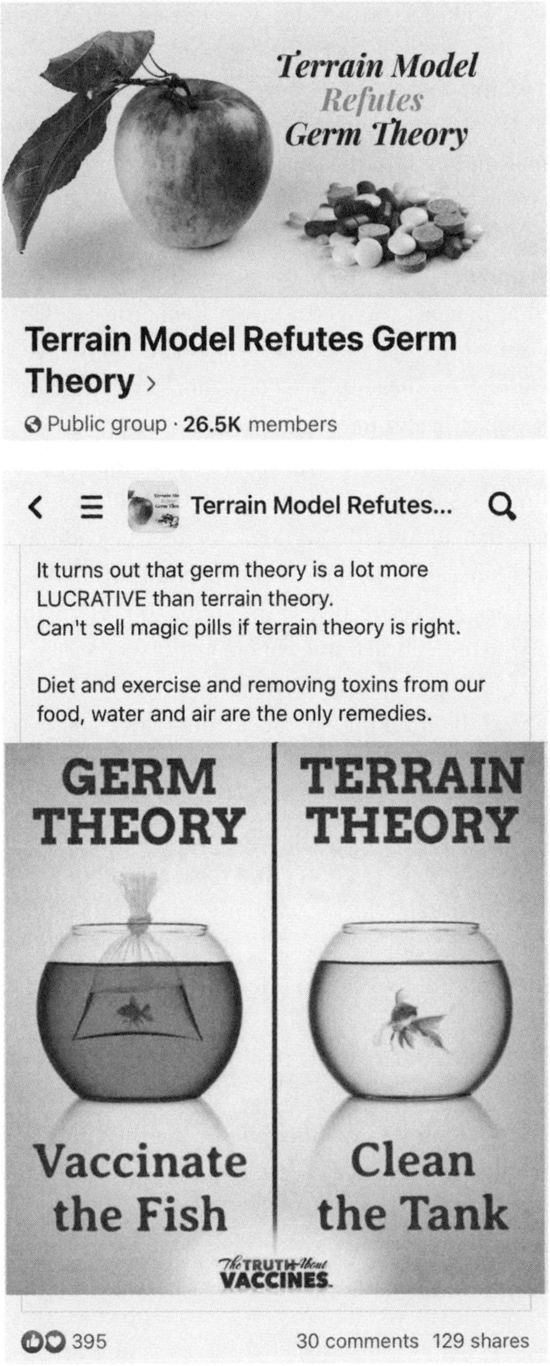

Figure 2.1 Screenshot photos of the Facebook group Terrain Model Refutes Germ Theory, dated August 30, 2022.

which supposedly illustrates the idea that terrain theory addresses health concerns with diet, whereas germ theory only requires pharmaceuticals. Another post claims that germ theory "is a lot more lucrative than terrain theory," which is consistent with Maher's statement that vaccination is "just a way to funnel money into the pharmaceutical companies." In Chapter 5 we will learn more about how these tropes—for example, "Treating the root cause" and "You're in the pocket of Big Pharma" (both of which are endorsed in Maher's statements)—are used to spread misinformation and propaganda.

It's not hard to imagine why germ theory denialism is a fan-favorite point of discussion among groups of people who share alternative medicine and anti-vaccine views: If one believes that germs don't cause disease, then it stands to reason that public health interventions aimed at preventing the spread of germs—such as masking and vaccination—are useless, and that alternative medicine treatments, such as unsupported supplements, "detoxes," and diet and exercise changes that address the "terrain," are the true pathways to health. It's no wonder that Maher, who parrots his talking points from these communities, has previously stated he doesn't "believe in vaccination." Germ theory denialism provides a unifying theoretical framework to justify such views.

We'll see later in this chapter that Maher has appeared to not have appreciatively advanced his thinking on vaccination since 2005. The problem is that his claims and similar views that deny germ theory are wrong—and not just simply wrong, but rather abysmally and jaw-droppingly wrong. Mounds upon mounds of overwhelming, high-quality scientific evidence supports germ theory. Despite Maher's contention that "a flu shot is the worst thing you can do," vaccination is widely considered to be among the greatest medical achievements of all time. According to the World Health Organization, vaccination prevents 3.5 to 5 million deaths every year from more than 20 life-threatening diseases, such as diphtheria, tetanus, pertussis, influenza, and measles. Worldwide data show that most vaccine-preventable diseases have been reduced to very low levels in many countries due to vaccination programs, which cannot be explained merely by the contribution of better hygiene and sanitation practices. Vaccination, then, is one of the closest things we have to a genuine medical miracle. It's not the high school biology textbooks across the world that are wrong; it's that the people who share Maher's views are failing to either understand or accept the science—or both.

* * *

Poor science literacy is a major problem. In a large U.S. national survey, only 64% of American respondents understood the statistical concept of probability, only 51% correctly defined a scientific experiment, and only 23% were able to correctly describe the components of a scientific study. And in the Facebook group "Terrain Model Refutes Germ Theory," it's probably a safe bet to assume that the majority of its over 26,500 members don't understand that germs cause disease.

Science literacy is a concept that has evolved over time, and it currently involves at least three related parts, according to the National Academies of Sciences, Engineering, and Medicine (NASEM), which is the collective scientific national academy of the United States. To be literate in science, we need to:

1. Possess knowledge about scientific content, such as knowing basic scientific facts, concepts, and vocabulary
2. Understand scientific practices, such as concepts related to hypothesis testing, probability, and correlation versus causation
3. Understand science as a social process, such as the role of peer review, the accumulation of accepted findings, and the nature of funding and conflicts of interest

Now, if you're like me, the idea of science literacy can feel daunting.

And yes, I have a master's of science degree and a PhD in clinical psychology, I publish research, and I'm even writing this book, which is about science. But science isn't easy! In graduate school, I once had an 8-hour-long exam in statistics, which I think might qualify as cruel and unusual punishment. While I passed the exam, I would almost certainly fail it today, as I haven't used those particular skills in quite a while. No one is perfectly versed in science literacy. In fact, even experts are experts only in a narrowly and highly specialized domain. But I must remind myself—and you—that becoming literate in science does not mean becoming an expert in science, which is an impossible task. Instead, to become literate in science means adopting the intellectual humility that is associated with the scientific spirit while at the same time constantly learning about science and finding a balance between trusting expertise and remaining skeptical about scientific claims.

Science Literacy Matters

I recently discovered a therapy called "Quantum Neurological Reset Therapy." If you search for it online, you will find a number of practitioners claiming that the therapy can be used to address both physical and mental health concerns, from early childhood trauma to chronic pain. It doesn't have a shred of credible scientific evidence to its name. According to the website of its founder, Dr. John Turner, a chiropractor, "Quantum Neuro Reset Therapy (QNRT™) is a proprietary protocol designed to initiate a quantum shift in the nervous system by resetting the brain's response to emotional triggers for both past and present emotional trauma and stress." If you didn't understand what that science-y sounding language means, it's because you're not supposed to. We'll learn more in Chapter 5—along with other pseudoscientific warning signs—about how such language is designed to confuse and deceive people with an end game of trying to sell products or services. The fact of the matter is that when you see the word "quantum" attached to any kind of therapy, you can be near certain that the therapy is a scam. The physicist and science communicator Richard Feynman has been popularly quoted as stating, "If you think you understand quantum mechanics, then you don't." Quantum mechanics is a highly complex, deeply counterintuitive, and fascinating area of physics—the obscurity of which lends itself perfectly to fake mental health experts who market their pseudoscientific wares through a haze of science-y sounding bullshit. Science literacy, in a sense, involves knowing just enough about quantum physics to understand that the alternative medicine practitioner trying to sell you a therapy apparently based on quantum physics doesn't understand quantum physics.

In other words, science literacy matters in part because it can help protect us against science-sounding fraudulent claims about our mental health. If we can learn how to gain just a basic understanding of scientific concepts and well-established scientific facts, in addition to pseudoscientific warning signs, then we are less likely to fall prey to the chiropractor, the self-styled wellness guru, or even the psychologist who nonsensically dresses up their brand of therapy in vacuous scientific jargon.

For example, I can recall the moment when my heart sank after a former patient of mine, Thomas, explained how he got duped by a local "integrative and functional medicine" clinic. It was our first meeting and I was conducting a psychological assessment to evaluate his mental health concerns. Thomas was experiencing severe posttraumatic stress disorder (PTSD). He had been enduring violent nightmares originating from his time serving overseas in the army. In that role, decades earlier, he had repeatedly stood within feet of pillage and murder, watching helplessly as innocent civilian families were destroyed in war. As he described those events, I shared in his heaviness as he wore tense mixtures of guilt, shame, and anger on his face. The years of nightmares had left him feeling depressed and suicidal. Part of my assessment involved taking a detailed treatment history. I learned that previous attempts to help him with psychiatric medications and eye movement desensitization and reprocessing therapy (EMDR) had fallen flat, and he had never received prolonged exposure therapy or cognitive processing therapy, two evidence-based treatments for PTSD (we will visit the nature of these treatments in Chapters 7 and 8).

A friend had suggested to Thomas that he contact the local integrative and functional medicine clinic given his lack of symptom relief. Thomas hadn't been employed for years due to his mental health difficulties, but he managed to muster nearly $2,000 to pay for a particular kind of light therapy called a Vielight in hopes that it would help. Light therapy does have some evidence to support its use for the treatment of seasonal and nonseasonal depression, and to a lesser extent PTSD. It usually involves around 30 minutes of daily exposure to a very bright light. Most studies involve therapies using a fluorescent lamp, which would typically cost you about $50 to $300. Scientists are still unclear about exactly why and how light therapy can work for some people.

That's not the impression you would get if you went to the website of the integrative and functional medicine clinic that sells the Vielight and markets the device for the treatment of PTSD (in addition to traumatic brain injury, concussion, Alzheimer's disease, Parkinson's disease, and the immune system). Without missing a beat, the website states that it works by "delivering photons to neuronal mitochondria which causes a cascade of beneficial cellular events/energy (ATP)." The Vielight is also not your run-of-the-mill fluorescent lamp. It's not even a lamp. It's a headset with wires and several ear-sized light-emitting diodes (LEDs) held in place on your head by two lateral stainless steel bands, as well as a diode that shoves up your nose, held in position by a plastic clip. It looks terribly uncomfortable. It's supposed to send pulsed near-infrared light to the brain though the skull and nose. Near-infrared light is a kind of light that we can't see because it lies outside the visible spectrum.

According to the website of the company that manufactures the Vielight, "Light therapy treatments, or photobiomodulation, has been a subject of heated debates and numerous attacks. Many skeptics and people distant from the science are questioning the benefits of photobiomodulation. Some of them out right rejecting the existence of the therapeutic benefits." Skeptics are correct to question the benefits of the Vielight because there's very little science to support its use—and virtually none for PTSD. The company website links to only one study related to PTSD, which is a case report showing improvements in pain and insomnia symptoms after using the Vielight among two war veterans who did not even meet diagnostic criteria for PTSD during the study. That's as far as the science goes.

To put it bluntly, Thomas was ripped off. He was sold a lousy science-y sounding product that he couldn't afford. He also told me it didn't work—and he was mad. Rightfully so. I wondered whether he would've purchased the product if he was more aware of just how crummy the evidence was that the Vielight rested upon, and just how classically pseudoscientific its advertising was.

When we take a bird's-eye view by looking at the scientific literature on science literacy itself, we discover that honing science literacy skills is a worthy pursuit. Studies have shown that people who exhibit lower science literacy skills are more susceptible to pseudoscience and misinformation in a variety of different topics related to science and health. For example, they're more likely to believe that the cure for cancer is being suppressed, or that childhood vaccines are unsafe and cause autism, or that people use only 10% of their brains, or that the alternative medicine treatment homeopathy can cure diseases. When people endorse such statements, they're endorsing a worldview that is not at all backed by evidence, which leaves them vulnerable to making health decisions based on inaccurate information.

Simultaneously, the complicated nature of our mental life never permits an easy, oversimplified story. You could have 10 scientific doctorate degrees and a Nobel Prize and still be duped by fraudulent claims and make poor health decisions. Science literacy matters in a dynamic sea of other factors that interact and influence our health decisions—which we'll learn more about in Chapter 6—such as how our minds are wired for mental shortcuts and thinking errors, how our prior beliefs can affect our reasoning, and how the social systems that we live in affect our ability to obtain quality information and health care. Sharpening our science literacy skills can help on all these fronts to embolden and protect us from misinformation and mental health scams.

Learning to Trust Expertise

Let's do a thought experiment: Imagine an alien comes to Earth and demands that you explain the concept of houses. That's easy for you, right? You've presumably stepped foot inside numerous houses throughout your life, as has everyone you know. Every time you go on a walk or drive, you see at least 50 of them. Explaining houses to aliens should be a piece of cake. And yet, as the alien takes a seat to listen, you realize you can tell him what a house is, but you can't explain much about them. How are they built? How did we as civilians come to live in houses? How are their prices determined? What are the laws surrounding them? How long have people lived in houses, and what did they live in before? Perhaps you can answer one or two of these specific questions, but surely the alien will have even more questions you can't answer. To think that housing is such a simple concept, and that you actually know much less than you'd predicted, puzzles you greatly.

That thought experiment is borrowed from the Decision Lab (http://thedecisionlab.com), which is a Canadian-based research firm devoted to elucidating and applying ideas in the field of behavioral science. The thought experiment illustrates a tendency that each of us leans toward, which is the belief that we understand more about the world than we really do. This tendency, known as the *illusion of explanatory depth*, is often not shattered until we are forced to sit down and explain knowledge we've always taken for granted. Leonid Rozenblit and Frank Keil coined the term in 2002 when at Yale University. They had research participants rate their understanding of everyday items—such as sewing machines, cell phones, and zippers—and then explain how the items worked. Following their explanations, participants rated their understanding of the items once again. Unsurprisingly, the second set of ratings was lower than the first.

A confession: I don't know much about some really important scientific topics, such as climate change, genetically modified foods, and nuclear power. But I don't feel embarrassed about my limited knowledge because I'm not a climate scientist, a biochemist, or a nuclear physicist. I don't have the ability to download to my brain the expertise that is painstakingly acquired over countless years of training and experience in those highly specialized fields. Admitting humility is better than the alternative of feigning expertise. In the 1930s, the British philosopher Bertrand Russell harshly declared, "The fundamental cause of the trouble in the modern world today is that the stupid are cocksure while the intelligent are full of doubt." To be fair, the harshness of his sentiment belies the fact that all of us are susceptible to overconfidence. But there's a lesson in there, which is that we are better off striving for a realistic view of our knowledge and to respect and learn from true expertise.

While knowing the basic facts established by science is one component of science literacy, it's a tall order! You might ask: Given that none of us can be experts in all scientific fields, what's the solution? I would offer that to become better versed in scientific topics we need to become familiar with scientific consensus, which refers to the leftover knowledge that has culminated and survived the gauntlet of everyday scientific scrutiny from countless experts around the world using the best available evidence. In other words, the scientific consensus is the most up-to-date, expert, scientific opinion that we have on various topics. It's true that uncertainty and incisive questioning are inherent to science and that a scientific consensus doesn't exist for every topic, but there are some topics on which consensus is clearer than others.

A 2022 study in the journal *Science Advances* asked people whether they agreed or disagreed with the scientific consensus on eight different topics:

- Climate change *(Consensus: Most of the warming of Earth's average global temperature over the second half of the 20th century has been caused by human activities.)*
- Genetically modified foods *(Consensus: Consuming foods with ingredients derived from genetically modified crops is no riskier than consuming foods modified by conventional plant improvement techniques.)*
- Nuclear power *(Consensus: Nuclear power is necessary and should be expanded to mitigate climate change.)*
- Vaccination *(Consensus: The benefits of vaccinations outweigh the risks, and vaccination has zero links to autism.)*
- Homeopathic medicine *(Consensus: There is no reliable evidence that homeopathic medicine is an effective treatment for any health condition.)*
- The Big Bang *(Consensus: The universe began approximately 14 billion years ago in a hot and dense state and has expanded and cooled since then.)*
- Evolution *(Consensus: Humans and other living things have evolved over time.)*

- Covid-19 *(Consensus: Measures such as social distancing and wearing a mask successfully reduce the spread of Covid-19.)*

The researchers found that no matter the topic, people who disagreed most with the scientific consensus knew less about it but thought they knew more. It would seem, then, that rejecting scientific consensus is a pretty good indicator of poor science literacy. For all their potential biases, flaws, imperfections, and conflicts of interest, it's still probably a better idea to trust in the collective findings of experts around the world rather than the musings of your neighbor or favorite uncle. Ultimately, not all opinions are equally valid when it comes to scientific expertise.

Thinking Scientifically

Science literacy involves much more than faith in scientific consensus, which we know can change over time. It's also about learning *how* to think, not *what* to think. If we "believe in" science, then we're doing it wrong. Science isn't a God. Or a unicorn. It's a tool to be used and a process to be understood. It helps to accumulate an evolving body of knowledge that is assembled within a sociocultural system. Teaching science as belief is, in essence, to teach pseudoscience. To learn how to think scientifically, we need to become familiar with how scientists actually do science.

It's beyond the scope of this book to detail the numerous ways that scientists wield their craft to explore and understand the natural world, including human experience. But some concepts are worth bearing in mind, particularly when it comes to informing ourselves about what treatments might be helpful for addressing mental health concerns.

In my experience with communicating science on social media, I've noticed one sticky line of thought that some people just can't seem to shake, which is the use of anecdotal evidence to support one's claims about the effectiveness of therapies. For example, you might hear someone proclaim: "I received Quantum Neurological Reset Therapy and my depression symptoms went away afterwards; therefore, it works." That's fantastic for them. But we must understand that their truth is not necessarily *the* truth. If their claim is to be used as evidence to support the treatment recommendations of other people, then we have a problem, as such a claim needs to be subjected to rigorous scientific scrutiny—for example, testing in randomized controlled trials (RCTs)—before any treatment can be recommended ethically by regulated mental health professionals.

Students of science will be familiar with the oft-quoted quip "The plural of anecdote is not data." The quip is a warning. It cautions that while personal health anecdotes are often a good starting point to generate research into the truth of health claims, the idea that anecdotal evidence confers low-quality scientific evidence is well established. An increasing number of anecdotes doesn't strengthen the quality of evidence, and many people can simply be wrong. In a post-truth era on social media, where literally anyone who has access to an account can voice a scientific opinion, the plural of anecdote is indeed not data, but risks becoming misinformation.

It's understandable why we all can fall victim to the illusory strength of anecdotal evidence. Our brains are readily tricked by one of the most powerful fallacies of human logic, known as the *post hoc, ergo propter hoc*. We commit this fallacy when we believe that because an event occurred first it must have caused a later event in question. But just because you take a shower every morning immediately before sunrise doesn't mean that your shower *causes* the sun to rise. Sometimes, two events are just correlated with one another coincidentally without one event causing the other. This illusion of causality, however, can be a stunning personal experience that tricks us into believing a false reality.

Some authors have even argued that illusions of causality lie at the heart of pseudoscience. I would further contend that the misuse of anecdotal evidence is the currency of alternative medicine, as providers in that community often capitalize on illusions of causality in the form of patient testimonials to advertise pseudoscientific treatments. With respect to psychologists, the use of patient testimonials in marketing materials and on websites is considered unethical, and even explicitly prohibited by several provincial regulatory bodies in Canada because it can result in this kind of inaccurate advertising, in addition to the fact that it could compromise the confidentiality of patients and exploit the inherent power imbalance that clinicians hold over patients. At the end of the day, anecdotal evidence is an unreliable way to determine the potential benefits and harms of therapies. Worse, anecdotes are often weaponized by those who are looking to promote a pseudoscientific agenda.

Thinking scientifically involves understanding how different kinds of evidence are weighted by scientists in their efforts to approximate the truth. Claims about health and treatments with little to no evidence behind them haven't been rigorously evaluated using the scientific method—instead, they may rely on weaker forms of evidence such as anecdotes, animal studies, or results from low-quality studies published in dubious journals that are inconsistent with a mountain of higher-quality studies and established scientific findings. In the world of mental health care, researchers and professionals use their judgment to differentiate credible scientific evidence from unreliable sources of information, and they loosely judge the merit of studies based on a hierarchy of evidence. I use the word "loosely" because, in fact, numerous versions of the hierarchy have been proposed and debated that take into account the idea that various kinds of studies each have their own strengths and weaknesses depending on the specific scientific question being posed. But to simplify things for the purpose of this book, Figure 2.2 shows a somewhat facetious version of the standard evidence hierarchy, where you can see that certain kinds of studies—for example, RCTs—are weighted higher than others. And no, YouTube videos, gut feelings, and health propaganda websites cannot be considered scientific evidence.

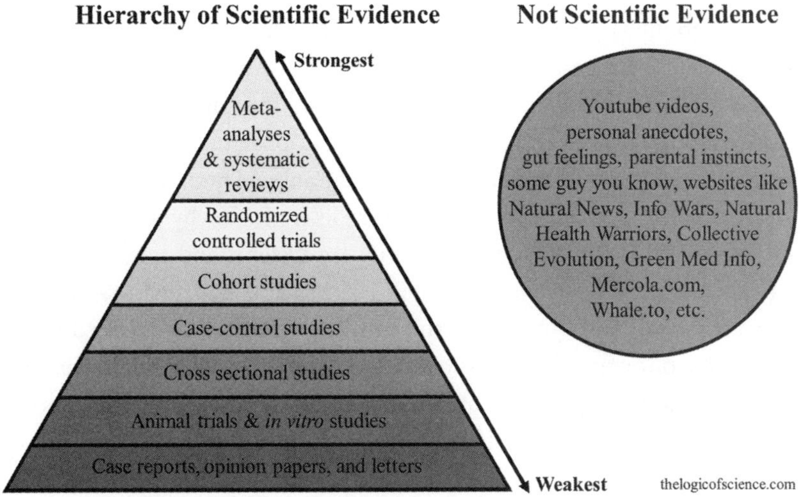

Figure 2.2 A somewhat facetious depiction of the hierarchy of scientific evidence versus its antithesis. By http://www.thelogicofscience.com
Source: http://www.mentalhealthliteracy.org

Science as a Human Endeavor

My friend Timothy Caulfield is a professor of health law and policy at the University of Alberta. You might recognize his name from his Netflix television documentary series, *A User's Guide to Cheating Death*, which was about debunking pseudoscientific myths in the wellness industry. It was an eye-opening show. He continues to devote his career to championing science literacy and to calling out grift, which has earned him both praise and scorn—a lot of scorn. As Caulfield put it:

> If you write about controversial stuff, you are bound to get a bit of hate mail. I get hate mail. Some of it is comprehensive ("I have yet to agree with any argument you have made about anything"). Some of it is pretty frivolous (there are people who really don't like my glasses). Some seems ideologically motivated ("M.A.G.A., Libtard!"). And some of it is beautifully succinct ("F*ck you, Timothy. Just f*ck you").

Experiencing hate mail and other serious forms of harassment can be tough on science communicators, but it sometimes comes with the territory. Caulfield handles it with grace and humor. Even better, like a true scientist, he learns from it. For example, he and his colleague once systematically analyzed the comments section from an article he wrote in the *Globe and Mail* about vaccination policy and the anti-vaccine rhetoric that can be found in the naturopathy community. After examining 330 comments made by 116 individuals, they found that, underlying the hate, one major theme emerged: mistrust—in researchers, physicians, pharmaceutical companies, the government, the "corporate" media, and Caulfield himself.

While some of the trust concerns were likely fueled by misinformation and conspiracies, lack of trust in health care systems and science per se is understandable. The scientific method is an antidote against the influence of our personal biases in our pursuit of truth—but it's also wielded by our inescapable humanity. Science is conducted by people, with people, in social structures, along with all our potentially conflicting and competing interests, motivations, desires, perceptions, emotions, and understandings. Trusting the scientific consensus can feel like blind faith.

It's not exactly obvious how research is prioritized and funded, how data are collected and analyzed, how the peer-review process works, how studies get published, how findings are communicated, how scientific consensus is reached, and how science is used to inform policy decisions. These messy, clunky, imperfect social processes of science were laid bare and buck naked for the public to see during the Covid-19 pandemic, as the world watched in real time how science was conducted. For some, it was unsettling and further fueled their mistrust in scientific institutions. For others, it helped improve their science literacy, as they learned that science doesn't occur in a vacuum but rather in a very social and political context.

Earning trust in science is imperative to improving public health and helping to combat the spread of misinformation. Learning how to think scientifically might even be easier for some people than learning to trust expertise in an environment where uncertainty, bias, and conflicts of interest coexist with the objective ideals and aims of the scientific method. Science literacy involves understanding the context in which science occurs with an eye toward trusting science that values research integrity and transparent science communication. Without these features, mistrust in science can be well earned and conspiracies driven by pseudoscience can become more attractive.

Your Other Friend: Mental Health Literacy

The year before I completed a PhD in clinical psychology, I spent 1 to 2 days per week in a hospital learning how to help people who experienced severe obsessive-compulsive disorder (OCD). I'm not referring to the colloquial, misunderstood use of OCD that we often hear in popular culture when people confuse it with meaning excessively neat, tidy, or organized, or when someone proclaims, "I'm so OCD." A person cannot be OCD—it isn't an adjective. I'm referring to the real deal: OCD is a mental disorder characterized by the debilitating presence of obsessions; that is, recurrent and persistent thoughts, urges, or images that are intrusive and unwanted, and/or compulsions, which are repetitive behaviors or mental acts that feel driven by obsessions or rigid rules.

The key word is *debilitating*. During those 1 to 2 days per week, I sat with people in both individual and group therapy sessions as they poured their heart out with respect to how OCD had stolen their lives. They would tell me, for example, how it should take them 10 minutes to drive home from work, but they would end up taking up to 8 hours to get home because every single time they hit a bump in the road, their OCD made them turn the car around to check whether they had hit a pedestrian. Others would tell me how they couldn't become intimate in relationships because they couldn't hug their partner out of an irrational fear that sperm would jump through their pants leading to pregnancy when their legs pressed against each other—they knew with 99.9% certainty that it was biologically impossible, but the 0.1% of doubt voiced by their OCD felt louder.

And still others would tell me how they couldn't even see or hear or touch the word "AIDS" on a piece of paper because their OCD made them feel it would increase their chances of contracting HIV—in a way similar to what they had read in Rhonda Byrne's best-selling book *The Secret*, which promotes the "law of attraction." The basic tenet of this law is that "like attracts like," meaning that if we want something in our lives, we simply need to focus our thoughts on that something and it will come to us. The law, of course, is scientifically ridiculous and often explained by its proponents through misrepresentations of quantum physics and other science-sounding or psychological-sounding language, such as "sending frequencies out to the universe." Its proponents are unsurprisingly silent about the darker side of its coin that implies people can also attract negativity and have the capacity to use their thoughts to pull themselves out of unjust treatment at the hands of poverty, racism, ableism, etc. Alarmingly, belief in the law can worsen OCD symptoms, as research has shown that a cognitive error called *thought–action fusion* occurs more frequently in the minds of people who experience OCD, as well as anxiety disorders. Thought–action fusion is the belief that simply having a thought about an event makes that event more likely to occur—for example, believing the thought "If I think about a car accident, it's more likely to happen." Not to be confused with the mental strategy sometimes used by athletes to visualize the motor movements in their upcoming performance, thought–action fusion is indistinguishable from the ridiculous law of attraction in any meaningful way.

As we sat in these therapy sessions together, we would develop meaningful therapeutic relationships and collaborate on solutions. Together, we would delve into the depths of their lives trying to gain a personalized understanding of the origins of the OCD and its current manifestation. Crucially, we would become coexperts on the nature of exposure and response prevention (ERP) and how to custom tailor the therapy to the unique way that OCD showed up for them. ERP is the best therapy available for OCD. As an advanced branch of cognitive-behavioral therapy (CBT), ERP sits atop a solid research foundation. Its essence involves volunteering to expose oneself slowly and safely over time to a variety of situations that trigger obsessions (i.e., "exposure") and then refrain from compulsions (i.e., "and response prevention"). The pace and intensity of the exposures are constantly negotiated depending on the patient's comfort level. It works because, over time, our brains are shown first-hand that we can cope with obsessions without responding with compulsive behaviors.

To an outsider gazing in, the therapy sessions can look interesting, to say the least. For example, I once sat in the passenger seat of my patient's car as we drove around the hospital parking lot purposely searching for visible bumps in the road to hit—we wanted to prevent checking afterward whether we had hit a pedestrian by not looking in the rearview mirror or getting out of the car. For the patients who were unable to hug their intimate partners due to fear of sperm jumping through their pants causing pregnancy, they were assigned exposure homework to consensually hug their partners with their pants on—and then off. They were also to refrain from their compulsions to wash their pants or shower afterward. And for those who were unable to see or hear or touch the word "AIDS," we would sit together on a laptop to challenge their thought–action fusion by intentionally and repeatedly typing the word "AIDS" and then physically touching the screen without sanitizing our hands.

Part of the therapy also involved laughing together at the absurdity of the work while acknowledging it as a necessary pathway to better health. It takes bravery to voluntarily jump into the deep end of the pool, so to speak, and to tolerate the discomfort associated with learning how to swim. It's certainly better than the alternative of being pushed in without consent. When engaging in ERP, I would bring the science, they would bring the art—in the form of self-knowledge—and together we would coexplore and create a plan. No therapy is perfect or can help everyone. But some, like ERP, work better than others, and we have the research to back that up.

More than 10 years later, I've tried my best to help countless others who've experienced the ravages of OCD, most often in the context of people seeking help with addiction concerns as well. When people experience mental disorders, such as OCD, it's understandable and not at all uncommon for us to want to alleviate that pain in ways that ultimately make it worse, such as with the use of psychoactive substances like alcohol that immediately but only temporarily drown out the noise. These substances should not be confused with the best psychiatric medications that we have available to treat

OCD—called selective serotonin reuptake inhibitors (SSRIs)—which often take a month or longer to begin working.

As patients came to see me, however, I was struck with disbelief, eventually turning to disappointment, time and time again, when I asked whether they had ever received ERP to help with their OCD. The answer was almost always a resounding "No. What's that?"

Some people had been suffering with OCD for years and even decades without ever being introduced to ERP, let alone receiving care from an ERP-trained mental health professional. I would ask, "Well, what kind of therapies have you received to address the OCD?" Many would reply: "Oh, you know, just like talk therapy, naturopathic and herbal stuff, and pills, and trying to eat differently." Some would even say that they've tried "CBT," but when I asked what that meant and involved, it became crystal clear that whatever they tried, it wasn't real CBT (which we'll learn about in Chapter 8).

As I continue to practice as a clinical psychologist, I still find myself wondering: Why have virtually none of my patients who experience OCD received ERP or been able to access it? Why haven't they even heard of ERP? Why aren't more professionals trained in ERP? Why are alternative medicine practitioners pretending they know how to help with OCD without any research to back it up? What is happening in the offices of some health professionals who claim to provide CBT that does not at all resemble CBT? And perhaps, most importantly, how can patients ensure that they're getting the best available care? In short: What gives?

* * *

Science literacy is foundational to mental health literacy. Without a firm grounding in scientific principles, understanding the science of mental health is an uphill battle. And like poor science literacy, poor mental health literacy is also a major problem. Studies have shown that mental health literacy among the public worldwide is low, as many people struggle to understand the nature of mental health and mental disorders, and many remain uncertain about how to obtain information and treatment if they encounter difficulties. Worse, worldwide studies have also shown that mental health literacy among health care professionals is not great either.

Mental health literacy involves understanding where our knowledge about mental health comes from. It also involves understanding how to actually *be* mentally healthy and how to seek professional help if needed. At its core, to be literate in mental health means to develop skills in at least four related areas:

1. Understanding how to obtain and maintain positive mental health
2. Understanding mental disorders and their treatments
3. Decreasing stigma related to mental disorders
4. Knowing when, where, and how to get help

Think of mental health literacy as a skill to be learned and practiced over time. No one pops out of the womb as literate in mental health. It's something we need to pay attention to and hone as new scientific information becomes available.

People with poor mental health literacy don't do well. A 2021 U.S. study found that American respondents demonstrated poor mental health literacy, as indicated by holding stigmatizing beliefs toward mental illness and being unable to identify mental disorder symptoms and appropriate courses of treatment. Those with poorer mental health literacy were more likely to say that they were experiencing higher rates of symptoms related to depression, anxiety, and stress, as well as feelings of stigma toward themselves. (The word "stigma" essentially refers to the bundle of attitudes and beliefs that contribute to people's fear, rejection, avoidance, and discrimination against particular ideas or groups—in this case, against mental illness and its evidence-based treatments.) Other studies have shown that people with better mental health literacy are more likely to both seek and use services to address their mental health concerns, whereas those with poor mental health literacy and negative attitudes toward mental health care, perhaps obviously, are less likely to engage with mental health services.

Poor mental health literacy has also harmed my own patients. For example, I can remember the first time that I heard about *kratom*—a dietary and herbal supplement—when a woman came to my clinic, reluctantly, seeking help to stop using it. Kratom derives from a plant called *Mitragyna speciosa* found in Southeast Asia and has rather unique psychoactive properties: In our bodies, physiologically, it acts as both an opioid and a stimulant, which means it can provide euphoria and relief from both pain and fatigue. In North America, its powdered leaves are usually consumed in a drink, but products and capsules marketed as containing kratom may also include contaminants—such as heavy metals and disease-causing bacteria—since it's an unregulated supplement. My patient had been purchasing her capsules online given that the sale of any product containing kratom is prohibited in Canada. In the United States, it can be purchased in some health food stores, vape shops, and even gas stations. Both Health Canada and the U.S. Food and Drug Administration (FDA) have issued warnings about its safety because side effects could include drowsiness, nausea, vomiting, seizures, liver toxicity, and excessively rapid heartbeat. It can also lead to addiction. In the past two decades, scientific reports have shown a dramatic increase in calls to poison control centers in the United States related to kratom, and many cases have required hospitalization resulting in serious medical problems.

My patient told me she began using kratom because she believed that as an herbal remedy, it was a "natural way" to treat her depression. She voiced a strong distaste for "pharmaceuticals and the medical-industrial complex," which steered her away from mainstream mental health care and toward alternative medicine options. Online forums and social media had led her to believe that kratom was a viable treatment for depression, with some people calling it "lifesaving."

Initially, the kratom worked—in a very loose sense of the word. It gave her the focus and energy she was lacking and numbed the intensity of her self-loathing thoughts. But none of these benefits lasted for long. After a few months of near-daily use, she needed to increase her dosages to feel the same effects. If she missed a day of using, then she would feel even more depressed on top of snappish irritability, uncontrollable diarrhea, painful body aches, wrenching nausea, and frustrating insomnia, which are classic opioid withdrawal symptoms. Her mind filled with thoughts of kratom and little else, until one afternoon, she overdosed. She was drifting in and out of consciousness, and barely breathing. Her boyfriend immediately drove her to the hospital where she was given naloxone, a medication to rapidly reverse the potentially lethal overdose.

In our therapy sessions together, my patient expressed feeling embarrassed for believing that "natural" plant-based opioids like kratom could be less harmful than synthetic or semisynthetic opioids like fentanyl or heroin, respectively. She regretted not seeking treatment sooner for her depression, noting that her long-held convictions and misperceptions about the evils of mainstream mental health care served as a barrier. Despite some harsh self-criticism, she arrived at an understanding that the kratom addiction she developed wasn't her fault, and she eventually overcame the internalized stigma she held against using opioid agonist therapies (OATs) to help treat the addiction, such as methadone or buprenorphine-naloxone (brand name: Suboxone). Fortunately, with psychotherapy and OAT, my patient was able to wean off opioids entirely and experience life again with zest and without the asphyxiating dark veil of depression.

Her fate could've been worse. For many people, it has been. The opioid crisis has caked the world in a layer of despair as overdose deaths have skyrocketed in the past two decades. From 1999 to early 2022, more than 600,000 lives were lost to opioid overdoses in North America—and researchers have estimated that an additional 1.2 million people will die due to overdose from 2022 to 2029. That's roughly twice the deaths in one-third the time it took the first 600,000 people to die. It's felt like an unspeakable curse to lose patients at our clinic, as well as a blessing to shake the warm hands of those who've made it through alive.

One patient in his 20s who became addicted to an illegally made version of the potent opioid *fentanyl* told me that he overdosed and was brought back to life with naloxone more than 10 times. He had never sought treatment before meeting with me. At our initial appointment, I asked him if he was scared to die. He replied that he was but elaborated that his fear of agonizing opioid withdrawal trumped his fear of death. When I asked what prevented him from seeking help sooner, he said, "I didn't think I deserved to."

Other patients too have told me they've avoided seeking treatment for similar reasons: They feel immoral, blamed, and stereotyped by the public as "addicts" or "junkies." Too much misinformation about the nature of addiction runs through our culture and seeps down to patients, such as beliefs that addiction reflects a moral failure or that people can just quit using if they try hard enough. The truth is that, by definition, addiction is characterized by clusters of psychological, behavioral, and physiological symptoms that lead a person to continue using *despite* the significant problems it causes themselves and others. Its impact is worsened when people feel shame and stigma rather than compassion.

In light of the opioid crisis and the misinformation and grift in circulation these days, it's unsurprising that scientists and health professionals are increasingly recognizing that we need to improve everyone's mental health literacy. It's much harder to fall victim to someone telling you that your depression can be cured with kratom if you understand exactly what depression is, how it's best treated, and how to find that treatment. It's much easier for people to seek treatment for opioid addiction when it's widely understood and its stigma is reduced.

To circle back, how much suffering might be spared too, for example, if people who experience OCD could identify their symptoms early, dodge the alternative medicine practitioner who pushes homeopathic products, for instance, and find a mental health professional who can competently provide ERP?

Science literacy and mental health literacy are tools of empowerment. You might not have control over the local availability of evidence-based treatments, but if you're equipped with science and mental health literacy, you're certainly better positioned to protect and advocate for yourself.

A Golden Ticket

> Please don't tan your butthole to treat your depression.
> Please don't detox from alcohol using unregulated supplements.
> Please don't let alternative medicine practitioners put ozone in your ear, your vagina, or up your bum.
> Please don't use essential oils to treat psychosis.

These are just some of the pleas I've given on social media. Sure, they might have a flair for the dramatic, but each was coupled with a real-world example that depicted the very "remedy" I was discrediting. On a daily basis, I am alerted to such examples by delving into the pseudoscientific trenches of the online world. Many people have asked whether I feel tired, or dismayed, or shocked as a result of feeling compelled to make these points. I will answer here: Yes, I feel all those emotions and more. At the end of the day, however, in our social media era, it's both my job and ethical duty to advance public understanding of mental health at a time when we really need it and in the very place where grifters grift. People are ravenously searching for ways to feel mentally healthy, and they are inundated by misinformation of this kind that can lead them astray.

Understanding how to obtain and maintain positive mental health is a key component of mental health literacy. It sounds like a golden ticket, doesn't it? We would all love to know exactly how to become and remain mentally healthy. But it raises a question that begs to be answered: What does it mean to be mentally healthy? Therein lies a philosophical minefield. Does mental health mean feeling good all the time? Does it mean never experiencing uncomfortable emotions? Does it mean the absence of a diagnosed mental disorder? Nope. None of those things.

If you scour the research literature, you will find many different definitions of mental health. My friend Senator Stanley Kutcher is a psychiatrist in Nova Scotia, Canada, and has been a long-time leader in helping people improve their mental health literacy through his government advocacy. He noticed that most definitions of mental health have one thing in common: They acknowledge that mental health is a reflection of a healthy brain.

This means that long gone are the days of what's called "Cartesian dualism," which is an idea proposed by the French philosopher René Descartes. Cartesian dualism describes the idea that the mind and body are totally distinct from one another. Converging and overwhelming evidence from numerous scientific fields indicates that this simply just isn't the case. Instead, the brain gives rise to the mind. In fact, they are so linked that it doesn't even make sense to consider them separately. Brain health is mental health, and vice versa.

Why does any of this philosophical mumbo-jumbo matter? It matters because it directly informs how we understand mental health. When my patients ask me what mental health means, here's what I tell them: Mental health doesn't involve the aim of eradicating uncomfortable emotions and life stressors. Rather, mental health involves practicing healthy ways to roll with, and grow from, life's punches. It involves a state of mental functioning in which a person can experience productivity, satisfied relationships, meaning and purpose, and high quality of life and possess the ability to cope with adversity. Stay tuned for Chapter 8, where we will take a deeper dive into the topic of what mental health really means.

Importantly, mental health and mental illness are not the same thing. Just as we can be physically healthy and still experience physical illnesses, we can also be mentally healthy and still experience mental illnesses. For example, a person can experience a mental illness, such as schizophrenia, and still experience mental health by regularly taking helpful medications, practicing healthy coping skills to manage symptoms and life stressors, and live their life with enjoyment and meaning.

Mental Illness Denial

Several years ago, I met Brandon. He was referred by his family physician to our clinic for help. He was a 24-year-old single White male who was living in a subsidized apartment and receiving unemployment income support. He had been fired from numerous labor jobs in the previous 5 years due to lateness and missing work. He told me that he tried to kill himself three times, most recently because he heard different voices in his head repeatedly disparage him and say that the world would be better off if he were dead. The voices would become thunderously loud after Brandon used cocaine and methamphetamine, but those drugs would give him the energy and motivation he felt he needed to combat his lethargy and leave his apartment to get groceries. Even during periods without drug use, he explained, he sometimes felt like his mind had been captured by repeating thoughts about people who were out to harm him. For example, he told me that whenever he saw coins on the ground, such as pennies, he believed it was a sign that a harmful person was near—and if he saw an arrangement of three similar objects in a triangle, such as three pennies on the ground, it was a message to flee immediately.

Brandon was no stranger to the emergency departments of a couple local hospitals, as sometimes he would go there voluntarily when he felt suicidal, and other times he was brought there, either by police or by his family, out of concern. Brandon's parents too were no strangers to the mental health care system in their frequent past and ongoing pursuit of help for their son. They told me that several psychiatrists had assessed Brandon over the years and said that he met diagnostic criteria for "substance-induced psychotic disorder" and, most recently, "schizophrenia," given that Brandon's psychotic symptoms—for example, his auditory hallucinations and delusional beliefs—occurred during times without drug use.

As I held therapy sessions with Brandon and his parents, it became tragically clear that misinformation was a threat to our treatment plan. When people are struggling with the chaotic intensity associated with schizophrenia, we know from the scientific literature and clinical practice guidelines that successful treatment involves many moving components with the use of both pharmacotherapy and psychosocial interventions. Antipsychotic medication is one such strong evidence-based component of treatment that can help target and ameliorate psychotic symptoms. Brandon's parents, however, were not fans of medication, to put it mildly.

They had read online that psychiatric medications shouldn't even be called "psychiatric medications" but rather "neurotoxins" that have a "poisonous" impact on the brain and mental life. They told me that in online forums, they learned not to trust "Big Pharma," which was suppressing the truth about how "natural" and "holistic" treatments with no side effects were healthier for their son. They even questioned whether mental illness existed in the first place because they had been sent several articles on social media about how the discipline of psychiatry is a dangerous fraud that "medicalizes" human suffering by inventing mental illnesses that are scientifically invalid. Brandon, not wanting to disappoint his parents and agreeing that Big Pharma was evil, told me that he felt mixed emotions about wanting to use medication, even though it had helped him in the past to find relief from his symptoms.

Brandon's case is not at all unique. Poor mental health literacy shows up frequently at my hospital clinic. It comes from a variety of sources, such as social media, popular culture, friends, and family. And it can interfere with a person's chances of receiving the best available care. In clinical practice, mental health professionals must be willing to navigate such misinformation in a way that adheres to evidence-based practice, respects patient autonomy, ensures safety, and empathically preserves therapeutic relationships. This delicate dance is no easy feat. One way to smooth the process for all parties involved is to raise the mental health literacy of the public, which in part involves becoming better versed in the nature of mental disorders and their treatments.

You're probably wondering: What exactly does mental illness mean? It's such a beast of a question that I've devoted the entire next chapter to its elucidation. In short, you might've noticed that mental health professionals will often use the terms "mental illness" and "mental disorder" interchangeably. And that's okay for now so that we don't get stuck in the weeds. Most of the time, when professionals refer to mental illnesses as mental disorders, they're referring to diagnosable conditions, such as those found in the *Diagnostic and Statistical Manual of Mental Disorders*, 5th edition, text revision (DSM-5-TR).

Some people like to refer to the DSM as the "Bible of Psychiatry." They're sorely mistaken. Allen Frances—a psychiatrist who was the head of the DSM-IV taskforce—often says something to this effect: "I equally distrust people who worship the DSM as those who ignore it altogether." This is because the DSM is more of a rough guide to the diagnosis of mental disorders than it is a rule of law, and it continues to be revised.

And it should continue to be revised! Mental health professions, such as clinical psychology and psychiatry, are scientific disciplines. Our understanding of the definitions and boundaries of particular mental disorders fluctuates over time, which reflects evolving scientific knowledge.

Mental disorders can be best understood as clusters of symptoms that cause significant distress and impairment to a person's everyday functioning. These clusters of symptoms co-occur in recognizable patterns that can be

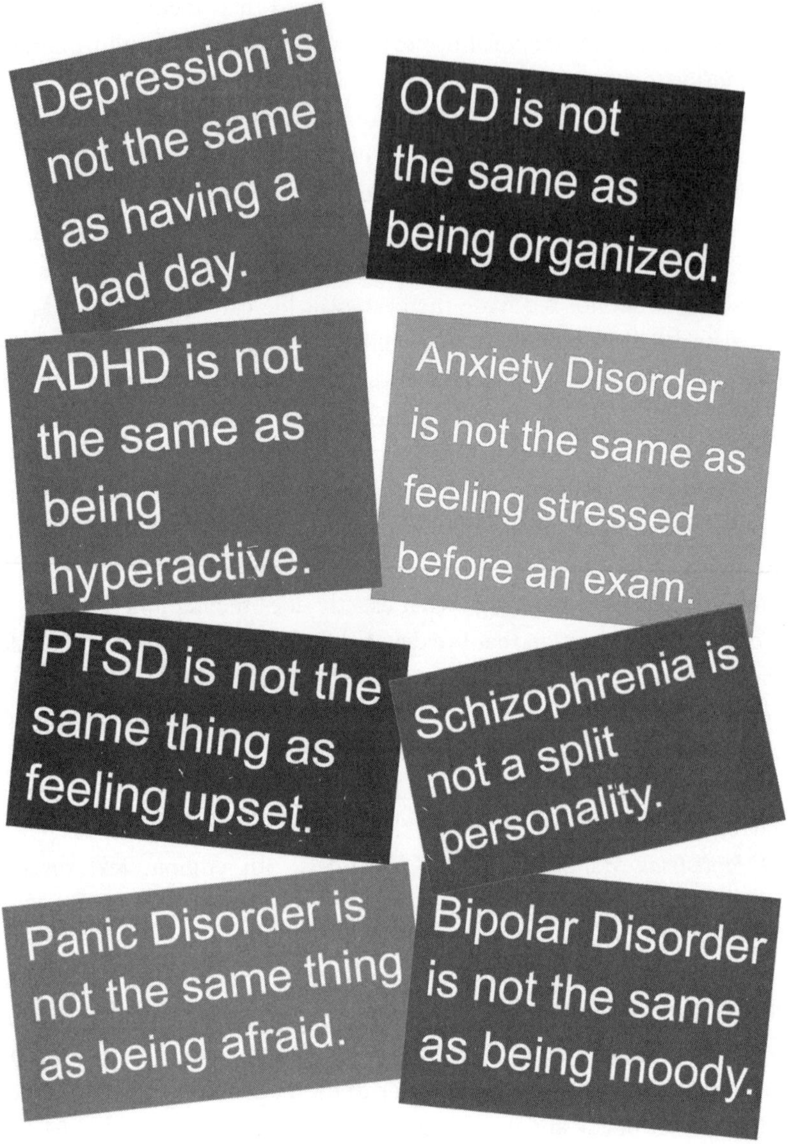

Source: http://www.mentalhealthliteracy.org

reliably identified. Mental disorder diagnoses can then be used as one important piece of information among many when deciding how best to help people and which evidence-based treatment approaches to draw from.

At the same time, evidence supports the idea that there's a continuum between mental illness and its absence. And the boundaries are not clear-cut. As the DSM-5-TR explains, "There is no assumption that each category of mental disorder is a completely discrete entity with absolute boundaries dividing it from other mental disorders or from no mental disorder."

I know the idea of fuzzy boundaries can feel deeply unsatisfying. But just as the unclear boundary between science and pseudoscience does not imply that the two cannot be meaningfully differentiated, the lack of discrete boundaries around mental illness does not imply that there is no such thing as mental illness or that the boundaries are completely arbitrary.

This shifting landscape isn't unique to mental disorder diagnosis either. The boundary between health and disease is fuzzy across all areas of medicine. For example, we don't hear anyone claiming that hypertension doesn't exist even though its determination is made by a somewhat arbitrary threshold. To quote psychiatrist Joe Pierre, "To say that mental illness isn't any one thing or that its definitional boundaries are fuzzy doesn't mean that it doesn't exist, anymore than we could credibly claim that the color *green* doesn't exist. The same could be said of planets, cars, or pain."

This topic might seem complicated, but that's because it is! Countless minds and careers have been devoted to trying to understand the nature of mental illness. Philosophical debates about how to apply precise terminology (e.g., illness vs. disorder vs. disease vs. condition vs. syndrome) rage on in the scientific literature across all medical disciplines. Mental health literacy involves becoming familiar and comfortable with this scientific uncertainty and complexity.

It also involves looking to bona fide mental health experts within their scientific communities to help lead the way to better understanding. Real patients and their families, such as those represented by Brandon's case, unnecessarily suffer when gripped by misinformation that outright denies the existence of mental illness, engages in fear mongering about the realities of medications, and stigmatizes psychiatric patients and their care along the way. Chapter 3 will take us on a journey to understand this kind of misinformation by going directly to its sources, which lie within the wellness community, anti-psychiatry movement, and mental health professions themselves.

The Invisible Bruise

I discovered Hannah Blum's inspiring work on Instagram. She is a writer, artist, and mental health advocate. And over a decade ago, she was diagnosed with bipolar disorder, which happens to be one of the most misunderstood experiences of mental illness.

I've noticed that many people mistakenly call themselves "bipolar" when they have mood swings during the day or difficulties managing their emotions. Bipolar disorder is neither of those things. The DSM-5-TR includes variations called *bipolar I* and *bipolar II disorder*. In short, people who experience bipolar I disorder typically have periods of clinically diagnosable depression lasting 2 weeks or longer, interspersed with periods of manic episodes. During these episodes a person feels like their mood is extremely and persistently elevated or irritable, and they have increased energy almost all day every day for at least a week—in that time they may barely sleep, be more talkative and impulsive than normal, have racing thoughts, and feel like their self-esteem has skyrocketed. People who experience bipolar I disorder typically have had trips to the hospital because their symptoms are so debilitating. Bipolar II disorder is similar but milder in its expression.

Blum uses art and poetry to educate and raise awareness about what it's like to live with mental illness, along with what it's like to feel shamed for it. One thing that caught my eye about Blum's work is the stigma she's faced from the wellness community.

"In the wellness space, people, including psychologists, produce content on social media that directly denies the existence of mental illness," she writes. "They shame people for taking medication. This is called *pill-shaming*. This is what kept me from taking my medication for years, which only caused more problems."

No one deserves to experience stigma for addressing their mental health needs—whether via psychotherapy, medication, or both. Research shows that when people feel stigmatized, it can lead to internalized shame and worsened mental health problems, and it can prevent them from seeking help—just as we saw above in the case of my patients who experienced opioid addiction.

When I spoke with Blum, she told me how she's felt stigmatized not only by pill-shaming but also by misinformation. She wrote, "A couple months ago, a family friend who is a spiritual healer and wellness coach told me that she could 'balance the bipolar out of me.'" As you might suspect, "balancing the bipolar" out of someone isn't a thing. Blum told me she considers this

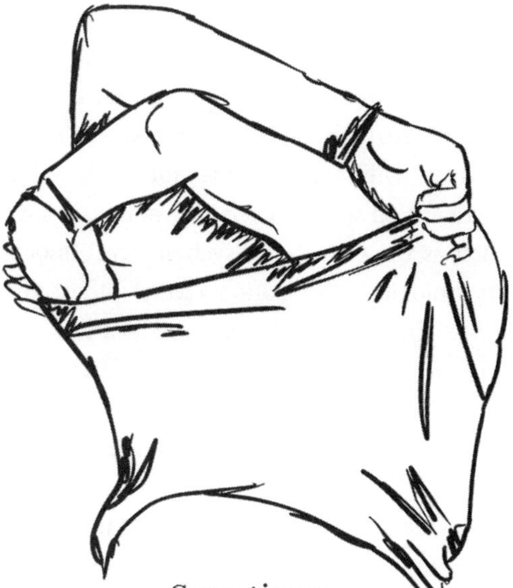

Sometimes,
I wish my mental illness
would show up like a bruise,
and I could say to the world,

"I told you it was real.
Now, maybe you'll listen."

kind of misinformation not only dangerous but also deadly, and it continues to motivate her advocacy.

Experiencing mental health concerns can be a heavy burden to bear alone. People fare much better mentally when they can offload, share, express, and ease that burden. As social creatures, we benefit when others become educated and help lighten the load.

Mental health literacy involves educating ourselves and others so that we can collectively decrease stigma. Again, my dear friend Senator Stanley Kutcher has wisely, throughout his career, been shouting from the mountaintops about the various ways we can all do this: We can seek out educational opportunities to learn more about mental disorders and their treatments. We can prioritize listening to those with lived experience. We can mind our language to ensure our use of terminology isn't perpetuating the very stigma we wish to avoid (e.g., not using derogatory terms such as "psycho," "crazy," and "junkie"). We can talk about our own mental health concerns to normalize the experience for others and show people that it isn't taboo. We can get active! This means using our voices and speaking up when we encounter mental health illiteracy in popular and social media. And we can exert our political power by supporting organizations—such as the Canadian Psychological Association (CPA) and the American Psychological Association (APA)—that advocate for public policies in the service of mental health science, education, and improvement.

Navigating the Wild West

Something happens when I go to parties—and it's not just my butchering of karaoke songs. Without fail, once people discover that I'm a clinical psychologist, they flock to tell me the mental health concerns experienced by their loved ones, or even themselves, and they ask me about the validity of various treatments and how to find good help.

A similar experience occurs on social media and via email. Strangers message me seeking information and guidance, sometimes with heartbreaking stories to tell. Ethically, if a person has not formally entered into a therapeutic relationship with me, then I am unable to help them beyond listening, empathizing, and pointing them to resources. It's tough.

The first step in getting good help is knowing how to locate and distinguish it from grift. It's so important that I've devoted Chapter 9 to unpacking that process. We know that when people feel less stigmatized and know where to look, they are better positioned to get the help they need. But where exactly can you find the resources you need?

There's a Latin term called *caveat emptor*, which translates to *let the buyer beware*. This phrase applies to seeking mental health services. It's an understatement to say that this is unfortunate. It's an outrageous reality. In any given jurisdiction, there can be a Grand Canyon–sized gap between the quality of mental health services that two people receive who present with the same mental health concerns. While this can obviously be the case for any service that a person receives—from restaurant service to brain surgery—it's a massive problem when it comes to the treatment of mental disorders.

This gap is so gaping not just due to variability among various mental health professionals in terms of their training and expertise but also because anyone can just set up a website or hang a shingle to promote themselves under a non–legally protected title such as "therapist" or "mental health clinician" or "wellness coach." For people to get good help, they need access to qualified, best-in-class mental health care from scientifically informed mental health professionals, such as clinical psychologists, social workers, psychiatrists, and nurses—and almost certainly not from their local alternative medicine clinic.

Getting useful mental health care is not easy. That's partly because there are cultural and system barriers that prevent quick and affordable access to evidence-based care, as well as the fact that it isn't immediately obvious where to look. While we all need to remain wary of people who really don't know what they're doing when it comes to trying to help someone with mental health concerns, there is also reason to remain hopeful. The good news is that there exist countless people who are well trained, ethical, and competent to deliver treatments that are indeed informed by science. But we desperately need to know how and where to find them.

In a perfect world, we would have an abundance of quality mental health services and easy and equitable access to those services for people from diverse economic and cultural backgrounds, and people would know exactly where to locate them. But then what? How do we know *when* to seek help? How do we know when our mental distress veers into the territory that requires the assistance of professionals? The reality is that there is no right or wrong answer to these questions.

Everyone could benefit from speaking to a well-trained mental health professional, and at the same time, not everyone needs or wants to. A useful indicator for when to seek help is to tune into your levels of distress and functioning. By distress, I mean your level of mental suffering. High levels of distress can be very normal reactions to life stressors, such as job or relationship loss or the death of a loved one. Mental distress alone doesn't necessarily mean that you're experiencing a mental disorder, and at the same time, that doesn't mean that you might not benefit from professional help. If you find that your levels of functioning have taken a hit too—for example, you're having trouble managing your responsibilities and everyday life tasks—then that could be your other cue to reach out. Mental health literacy involves prioritizing and dialing in to your mental health needs.

* * *

Seventeen years after Bill Maher appeared on CNN's *Larry King Live* deriding the flu shot, he made an appearance on *The Joe Rogan Experience* podcast in 2022 to voice his displeasure with Covid-19 vaccines. This statement perhaps best summed up his consistent anti-vaccine views and captured both his mistrust and disdain for public health officials:

> We are perfectly certain that this vaccine is safe! You don't fucking know that!

That mistrust and disdain was once again made even more apparent when in 2023 on Maher's own podcast, *Club Random With Bill Maher*, he interviewed then–presidential candidate and anti-vaccine activist Robert F. Kennedy Jr., stating:

> There's this idea we have in this country that we can avoid germs. It's not healthy. . . . You're fighting against something very powerful, which is [people's] health. They're super scared. So what do people do when they're scared? They create this idea that there's this safe place. And what is the safe place? Western medicine. Doctors. If someone has a white lab coat on, they think God is talking. That's the problem with *the science people*. You know, the ones wearing masks alone outside. Still. These morons. When they say *the science*, that's when you lose me completely.

While the conflicting and in some cases botched messaging from public health officials that occurred during the pandemic undoubtedly fueled Maher's mistrust, and that of the public, no scientist worth their salt would declare perfect certainty with respect to scientific claims, as the scientific method involves a tentative and humble process. Like all vaccines, Covid-19 vaccines went through a rigorous, multistage testing process, which included large clinical trials involving tens of thousands of people, specifically designed to identify safety concerns. Even back in 2022, literally billions of people had been safely vaccinated against Covid-19 according to the World Health Organization. Monitoring of Covid-19 vaccine safety is an ongoing scientific endeavor. Data collected from around the world make it clear that the benefits of Covid-19 vaccines outweigh the potential risks, including, in rare cases, serious adverse health events.

I've tried to make the case in this chapter that honing our science and mental health literacy skills matters for our own mental health and public health. And simultaneously, that it isn't enough. While Carl Sagan argued in 1995 that pseudoscience is embraced in exact proportion as real science is misunderstood, we now know that pseudoscience and misinformation are driven by more than just a lack of literacy skills. More variables need to be entered into Sagan's equation, as we'll see in Chapter 6, such as the influence of our biases, thinking errors, prior beliefs, motivations, and social systems.

People will still deny germ theory. And the existence of mental illness. They will still argue that the Earth is flat, gravity is an illusion, and evolution is wrong. Some people will remain unreachable. Others, perhaps with some guidance, will free themselves from the shackles of their deeply held, albeit profoundly pseudoscientific, beliefs. Your job is to stay the course and keep learning.

3

Crash Course in Psychopathology

One of the world's highest-paid actors, Tom Cruise, appeared on Matt Lauer's NBC *Today* morning show on June 24, 2005, to promote his blockbuster movie *War of the Worlds*. It was an infamous and heated interview that would have the internet talking decades later, in part because it showcased Cruise's disdain for psychiatry. And it wasn't the first time. Weeks earlier, Cruise had appeared on the television show *Access Hollywood* and chastised fellow actor Brooke Shields, calling her "irresponsible" for using antidepressant medication to treat postpartum depression. When Lauer questioned Cruise about his comments toward Shields, Cruise went on the offense:

CRUISE: I've never agreed with psychiatry, ever. Before I was a Scientologist, I never agreed with psychiatry. And when I started studying the history of psychiatry, I understood more and more why I didn't believe in psychiatry. And as far as the Brooke Shields thing is, look. You gotta understand, I really care about Brooke Shields. I think here's a wonderful and talented woman. And I wanna see her do well. And I know that psychiatry is a pseudoscience.

LAUER: But—but Tom, if she said that this particular thing helped her feel better, whether it was the antidepressant or going to a counselor or psychiatrist, isn't that enough?

CRUISE: Matt, you have to understand this. Here we are today where I talk out against drugs and psychiatric abuses of electric shocking people, okay, against their will, of drugging children with them not knowing the effects of these drugs. Do you know what Adderall is? Do you know Ritalin? Do you know now that Ritalin is a street drug? Do you understand that?

LAUER: The difference is . . .

CRUISE: No, no, Matt.

LAUER: This wasn't against her will, though.

CRUISE: Matt, Matt, Matt, Matt . . .

LAUER: But this wasn't against her will.

CRUISE: Matt, I'm asking you a question.

LAUER: I understand there's abuse of all of these things.

CRUISE: No, you see. Here's the problem. You don't know the history of psychiatry. I do.

LAUER: Aren't there examples, and might not Brooke Shields be an example, of someone who benefited from one of those drugs?

CRUISE: All it does is mask the problem, Matt. And if you understand the history of it, it masks the problem. That's what it does. That's all it does. You're not getting to the reason why. There is no such thing as a chemical imbalance.

LAUER: So, postpartum depression to you is . . .

CRUISE: Matt . . .

LAUER: Kind of a . . .

CRUISE: Don't.

LAUER: Little psychological gobbledygook . . .

CRUISE: No. No. I did not say that.

LAUER: I'm just asking, what would you call it?

CRUISE: No. No. Now, you're talking about two different things.

LAUER: But that's what she went on the antidepressant for.

CRUISE: But what happens, the antidepressant, all it does is mask the problem. There's ways of vitamins and through exercise and various things. I'm not saying that that isn't real. That's not what I'm saying. That's an alteration of what I'm saying. I'm saying that drugs aren't the answer, these drugs are very dangerous. They're mind-altering, antipsychotic drugs. And there are ways of doing it without that so that we don't end up in a brave new world. The thing that I'm saying about Brooke is that there's misinformation, okay. And she doesn't understand the history of psychiatry. She doesn't understand in the same way that you don't understand it, Matt.

One week later, Shields penned an op-ed in the *New York Times*, decrying Cruise's comments, not just for own sake but also "for the hundreds of thousands of women who have suffered from postpartum depression." She stated: "While Mr. Cruise says that Mr. Lauer and I do not understand the history of psychiatry, I'm going to take a wild guess and say that Mr. Cruise has never suffered from postpartum depression."

Ironically, Cruise's diatribe was riddled with misinformation and antipsychiatry tropes. Research shows that antidepressant medication can be helpful for postpartum depression, and as a general statement, they're safe, not "dangerous." They're also not "antipsychotic drugs," which are actually a different class of evidence-based medications used to treat psychotic disorders. Stimulant medications, such as both Adderall and Ritalin, are not "street drugs" used to "drug children" but rather can be helpful for attention-deficit hyperactivity disorder (ADHD). And despite more of Cruise's fear-mongering rhetoric about "psychiatric abuses of electric shocking people against their will," electroconvulsive therapy (ECT) is a safe, evidence-based treatment for severe mental illness. If you take a tour of a psychiatry inpatient unit at a hospital, you will see that it's not at all like how it's violently and inhumanely depicted in movies, such as the iconic *One Flew Over the Cuckoo's Nest* (1975), in which Nurse Ratched uses ECT as a threat to subdue people. Today, ECT is given to people under anesthesia when they're asleep, like a minor surgery, and only to patients under very specific circumstances, such as life-threatening severe depression. Perhaps most importantly of all, modern psychiatry is not a pseudoscience but rather embraces a philosophy of evidence-based practice in its codes of ethics and legal standards of practice.

If we take a step back, we can see that misinformation derived from anti-psychiatry ideas has infiltrated popular culture, from outspoken celebrity Scientologists like Tom Cruise, John Travolta, Danny Masterson, and the late Kirstie Allie voicing anti-psychiatry views in the media to on-screen depictions of psychiatric horror, such as the movie *Shutter Island* (2010) and TV series *American Horror Story: Asylum* (2012). In April 2022, even billionaire Elon Musk tweeted to his over 90 million followers at the time: "Wellbutrin is way worse than Adderall imo. It should be taken off the market. Every time that drug has come up in conversation, someone at the table has a suicide or near suicide story." Incidentally, research reveals that Wellbutrin, also known as bupropion, has helped many people who experience depression and some with ADHD, with at least one meta-analysis of randomized controlled trials showing that it does not increase suicidality.

Where does this kind of misinformation come from? To understand anti-psychiatry views, we need to better understand what it means to experience and treat mental disorders, which if you recall from Chapter 2 is one component of mental health literacy. Once we're equipped with a firmer grasp on the science of psychopathology, we can then counter misinformation with a critical lens by tracing it to its various sources in the wellness community, anti-psychiatry movement, and mental health professions themselves.

Crazy or Insane? What's in a Name?

Have you ever wondered if you're normal? What about crazy or insane? What do people mean by these terms: "normal" versus "crazy" versus "insane" versus "lunatic"? While the *Merriam-Webster Dictionary* may provide some answers to understanding these everyday colloquial terms, it doesn't do a great job at answering some more complex definitional questions, such as the difference between "mental health" versus "mental illness." The distinction between those terms eludes us in part because it's rooted in the very convoluted history and evolution of modern-day psychiatry.

We learned in Chapter 2 that defining concepts such as mental health and mental illness is complicated, but it's not for lack of trying. Philosophers, psychologists, psychiatrists, anthropologists, and other social scientists and medical professionals have all had their say, way back to ancient civilizations before such professions were formalized. It was in the late 19th and early 20th centuries that the effort to describe and classify mental illness really accelerated.

In fact, the roots of our current understanding of mental illness can be traced to 1856. Yes, a single year, because that's when two human pillars of modern psychiatry were born, only 3 months and 300 miles apart: German professor of psychiatry Emil Kraepelin and Austrian neurologist Sigmund Freud. Kraepelin's contribution to our collective understanding involved efforts to devise a classification system for mental illness based on very careful clinical observations of his patients and the trajectory of their symptoms. Around the same time, the rise of psychoanalysis, founded by Freud and his like-minded company, also began to dominate discussions and interpretations of what it means to be mentally ill. Psychoanalysis was a very different kind of theoretical system for understanding mental illness from Kraepelin's. It involved interpreting symptoms as clues to unconscious conflicts within the minds of patients, whereby the central aim of psychotherapy was to uncover and resolve those conflicts.

Psychoanalysis essentially blotted out Kraepelin's classification vision for the next half-century. Most of Kraepelin's scientific contributions in Europe failed to be influential in the United States at that time. This is a big deal because the United States is the birthplace of the *Diagnostic and Statistical Manual of Mental Disorders* (DSM). Recall from Chapter 2 that the DSM is sometimes mistakenly called the "Bible of Psychiatry" in popular culture because it's widely used today to help guide diagnosis and treatment of mental illness—it isn't meant to be used religiously. In the early days of American psychiatry, Freudian psychoanalysis reigned supreme; consequently, the beginning of the DSM series was heavily based on psychoanalytic ideas, from the DSM-I in 1952 through the DSM-II in 1968. For instance, in the DSM-I, disorders were described using succinct, vague language with no criteria for diagnosis and often laden with psychoanalytic terminology (e.g., "schizophrenic reaction").

Then, in 1980, the series changed focus: The DSM-III turned sharply away from psychoanalytic theories and purposely aligned itself with the rest of the medical world by reintroducing Kraepelinian ideas to understand mental illness. This meant that psychiatry was once again adopting a view of mental illness that could be understood like other medical disorders, with accompanying clinical signs, symptoms, and course over time, which would provide a much easier foundation for scientific research on the causes, prevention, and treatment of mental illness. This pivot was called the *neo-Kraepelinian revolution*. And it was successful insofar as it allowed clinicians of diverse theoretical persuasions to reliably agree about whether they were witnessing the presence of a particular disorder in their patients even if they disagreed about its causes or optimal treatments. It also set the stage for an explosion of meaningful research on the biological, psychological, and social aspects of psychopathology, leading to the identification of the best evidence-based treatments we have for specific disorders using randomized controlled trials.

That success, however, needs to be grounded in the sobering reality that the DSM is like a terrible map. Clinicians and researchers rightfully complain that it fails to accurately carve nature at its joints, so to speak. For example, the number of DSM disorders has approximately tripled from around 100 disorders in the DSM-I to around 300 in its current iteration, the DSM-5-TR. This means that while the DSM allows clinicians to reliably diagnose individual disorders, it has also increasingly expanded the range of conditions we consider to be a mental disorder, so much so that studies have estimated that about one-half of Americans will meet criteria for a DSM disorder at some point in their life.

This idea, of expanding the meaning and use of a psychological term to the point that its definition changes, is known as *concept creep*. If you stop and reflect on how certain psychological terms have been used in popular culture over the years, then you might notice the phenomenon occurring, for example, in how we colloquially talk about *abuse*, *bullying*, *trauma*, and *addiction*. In the case of mental disorders, the risk is that creeping definitions inadvertently end up "medicalizing" ordinary emotional distress. This is a valid concern because the insidious expansion of what it means to experience a mental disorder can lead clinicians to overdiagnose psychopathology and overprescribe medications when they aren't warranted. On the other side of the coin, defining mental disorders so broadly can beneficially normalize the idea that even some ordinary forms of emotional distress are incapacitating and warrant clinical attention.

While the DSM is terrible for navigation, it's still the most user-friendly map we have for describing mental illness—and in the remarkably imperfect and difficult science of psychopathology, that's better than no map at all. Just think: Our brains are home to an average of 86 billion neurons that communicate in ways we don't fully comprehend and are responsible for everything about our human experience, from how we feel love and conceptualize our personal identity to how we see objects and breathe without trying. It would physically take us almost 32 years to even count to 1 billion—assuming a counting rate of one number per second—because the number is that large. Multiply that by 86 and the complexity of the brain leaves scientists working tirelessly in their laboratories, slowly pushing our understanding forward.

Sure, it's easy to chastise the DSM, and it should be chastised, because that's how science proceeds. A waning enthusiasm for the DSM has been felt among both clinicians and researchers for decades. The current scientific literature pits multiple models of psychopathology against each other. It's beyond the scope of this book to break down these nuances, but here's a flavor.

Broadly speaking, three approaches exist as the frontrunners to describing mental illness. The first is the neo-Kraepelinian view now used in the DSM, otherwise known as the *categorical approach* to psychopathology. This is the view that is most often used in clinical practice, and it suggests that observable signs and subjective symptoms of mental disorders cluster together in recognizable patterns reflecting an underlying disease entity. As we learned in Chapter 2, however, even the DSM itself concedes that there exist fuzzy boundaries between different mental disorders and also between having or not having any mental disorder at all.

The existence of these fuzzy boundaries has given rise to a second approach to describing mental illness, the *dimensional approach*. It argues that the reason signs and symptoms of mental disorders reliably cluster together in patterns is not due to an underlying disease entity per se, but rather due to combinations of underlying dimensions that can be used to describe our mental life. For example, while you could be described as being either an extraverted or introverted person, it's richer to describe this one dimension of your personality as lying on a continuum, whereby you're more or less extraverted compared to others. The categorical and dimensional approaches agree that signs and symptoms don't cluster together randomly, but they disagree about why this happens.

The third approach to describing mental illness is called the *network perspective*. This is newer and radically different from its predecessors, the categorical and dimensional approaches. The network perspective doesn't view mental disorders as reflective of underlying disease entities *or* combinations of latent dimensions; it instead offers the idea that the relationship between various signs and symptoms *is the disorder itself*. For example, when one experiences addiction to alcohol, certain patterns between signs and symptoms become predictable. A person may experience anxiety in social situations, which motivates them to use alcohol when leaving their home, and in turn, over time, it results in the development of physiological dependence on alcohol. In essence, network perspectives allow researchers to understand mental disorders as a dynamic system of symptom-to-symptom interaction.

I'm going to pause for a moment because I know this material might seem super dense and difficult to understand. As an adjunct assistant professor, I've sat on plenty of academic committees, and I can assure you that even the most astute doctoral students of clinical psychology and exceptional faculty members have difficulty mastering these concepts. The point is that the science of psychopathology is supposed to be hard. It's advancing, as it should, and with that progress comes new understanding.

The scientific consensus may reach a point in the near future where it moves even further away from the DSM, not only in research settings, but also in clinical practice, where almost 90% of psychologists say they regularly, albeit lukewarmly, consult the DSM. Some mental health professionals will say we're already at that point, and some research in fact shows that other kinds of clinicians, such as physicians, don't tend to rely on the DSM for diagnosis. In my own clinical practice—working with and among psychologists, psychiatrists, other physicians, nurses, nurse practitioners, social workers, and occupational therapists—I see and experience first-hand how the DSM can be a clinically useful tool in some instances and be entirely useless in others.

We are collectively learning more every day about how to better describe psychopathology and what causes it in the first place. When people come to treatment for mental health concerns, they want to know about what ails them. It's normal to want to know exactly what's the cause of suffering and how to make it go away. The causes of psychopathology are as complex as pinning down a diagnosis.

In the field of developmental psychology, two fundamental principles called *equifinality* and *multifinality* neatly illustrate this complexity. Equifinality means that a mental disorder can arise as the result of the interaction between many different genetic and environmental factors. In other words, two people with different genetic profiles and different personalities and different upbringings can both experience the same mental disorder. For example, if you attend an Alcoholics Anonymous meeting, you will meet people from all walks of life, some of whom are victims of childhood abuse, and some who would describe a fantastic childhood. The Italian proverb "All roads lead to Rome" is based on the fact that in the days of the Roman Empire, the roads literally radiated out from its capital city in the center of the empire. The proverb means that there are many ways to get to the same place—that's equifinality.

In contrast, multifinality refers to the opposite process. It means that one common factor can lead to the development of multiple different mental disorders. Let's keep with the example of childhood abuse. Some people who experience childhood abuse will go on to develop posttraumatic stress disorder, whereas others might instead develop an addiction to alcohol, a persistent depressive disorder, schizophrenia, or no disorder at all. These principles underscore just how individualized the causes of our own mental suffering can be.

Good clinicians will provide a space to get to know you and your story where you're free to say anything and everything you wish. Together, you'll collaborate and co-explore how to best understand and address your mental health concerns. Good clinicians will have a basic understanding of the science of psychopathology and will communicate honestly. They will acknowledge the current state of the science, its limitations, and the fruits of what it has to offer. They won't dupe you or offer pseudoscientific assessments and treatments. And they certainly won't misinform you about the history and current status of psychiatry.

The Anti-Psychiatry Movement

In graduate school, one of my professors assigned an article to read that blew me away. It was written in 1960 and titled "The Myth of Mental Illness" by psychiatrist Thomas Szasz. It began by stating, "My aim in this essay is to raise the question 'Is there such a thing as mental illness?' and to argue that there is not." The idea of mental illness denial was a foreign concept to me at the time. Here I was, in graduate school, scrambling to learn the science of psychopathology by reading about it all day, every day. I was attending practicum placements at hospitals as my first professional foray into seeing mental illness with my own eyes. And then this article by Szasz comes across my desk and purports to undermine what I had been learning and witnessing first-hand. At that time, I didn't get it and was confused. Yes, I understood that our theories and models of psychopathology were incomplete and evolving, but I couldn't understand how people—let alone psychiatrists and other mental health professionals—could not believe that mental illness existed.

So I decided to dig further. I discovered that Szasz published a book in 1961 by the same name, *The Myth of Mental Illness*, as well as numerous others. I dove into some of these works and was jaw-dropped again by another piece of prose that he wrote over 30 years later, in 1996:

> I believe viewing the schizophrenic as a liar would advance our understanding of schizophrenia. What does he lie about? Principally about his own anxieties, bewilderments, confusions, deficiencies, and self-deceptions. He pretends that he is not confused, impotent, and insignificant; he is confident, powerful, and supremely significant.

You'd be hard pressed to find a more inaccurate and stigmatizing statement than that toward people who experience schizophrenia—a debilitating mental disorder characterized by combinations of psychotic symptoms that could include delusions, hallucinations, disorganized speech, catatonia, and avolition. My capacity for surprise took yet another blow when I learned that one of my favorite philosophers of science, Karl Popper, wrote a letter to Szasz in 1961 calling *The Myth of Mental Illness* admirable and fascinating, and stating: "It is a most important book, and it makes a real revolution." What was going on here?

I didn't know it at the time, but it *was* a revolution. Popper was right. Szasz had in part sparked a counterrevolution known as the anti-psychiatry movement. He was joined in his efforts by other psychiatrists, now heroes of the movement, including R. D. Laing, Franco Basaglia, and David Cooper, who coined the term "anti-psychiatry" in 1967 after the movement had already begun. The French philosopher Michel Foucault was also one of its intellectual pillars, as he wielded and wove together perspectives from sociology, anthropology, and history to critique psychiatry as an institution.

What were they rallying against? They were pushing back against psychiatry's dark past. They had a right to be angry. The movement was motivated by animosity toward psychiatry's history of inhumane asylum care, inappropriate pathologizing of minority groups, and perceived arbitrariness of diagnosis.

And it worked. The movement helped propel reform and pushed the discipline toward a more scientific endeavor. Psychiatry got its act together through rapid deinstitutionalization, closing many psychiatric hospitals and shifting patient care to regular hospitals and in the community and at home. The neo-Kraepelinian revolution embodied in the DSM-III greatly improved diagnostic practice. And a lively focus on the interaction between biological, psychological, and social contributions to mental health and illness—known as the biopsychosocial model—became adopted by psychiatry and helped smooth relations between clinicians with different theoretical orientations. As a result, by the early 1980s, the anti-psychiatry movement had diminished dramatically.

It didn't die, though. It transformed and lost its way. While modern psychiatry adapted and survived by aligning itself with the scientific spirit, modern anti-psychiatry—a disorganized movement existing largely outside of the medical world—became a pseudoscientific smorgasbord of misinformation. Scientific criticism is now a built-in feature of psychiatry, and it's healthy and paramount for the growth of the discipline. That's not what modern anti-psychiatry offers. Instead, it aims to tear down the discipline and deter treatment seeking. Much like the anti-vaccine movement, its criticisms toward psychiatry are moralistic and ideological, and not scientific, but rather pseudoscientific, as its messages are most often found on social media and in non-peer-reviewed sources, such as blogs, books, and opinion articles hosted on websites dedicated to flaming psychiatry in a way that dodges scientific critique. The movement has outlived its cause.

The decentralized lifelines of anti-psychiatry are given breath from a few different sources: fringe scholars, consumers, and members of the Church of Scientology. All tend to resent or reject the term "anti-psychiatry," which, incidentally, is not unlike the attitude of those who feel offended by the term "anti-vaccine" but nonetheless actively participate in the anti-vaccine movement by regularly creating or amplifying its content.

In academia, anti-psychiatry views find their expression in the Trojan horses of "critical psychiatry" and "critical psychology." These are subdisciplines composed of disgruntled psychiatrists and psychologists, as well as other scholars and journalists who base their work on critical theory, a broad philosophical approach to understanding topics through the lens of cultural assumptions, social structures, and power dynamics. Most of the insights offered are not new or beyond which psychiatry has already acknowledged and incorporated within its own biopsychosocial lens, such as the urgency to move toward a more humanistic model of patient care and away from a siloed focus on biology and pill dispensing. Such authors often have limited real-world clinical experience helping people with severe mental illness or collaborating with psychiatrists. Also, it just so happens that many of them have found fame and fortune basing their careers around anti-psychiatry stances.

Outside of academia, anti-psychiatry has paralleled the footsteps of the anti-vaccine saga in transforming into a grassroots, consumer movement composed of patients who identify as being harmed by psychiatry and those sympathetic to their cause. Its incarnations can mostly be seen through internet activism in devoted blogs, websites, YouTube channels, and social media pages. A cursory search will readily reveal notable examples of YouTube videos in the vein of "Psychiatry Exposed!" (over 134,000 views), TikTok hashtags related to #psychiatryharms (over 284,000 views) and #antipsychiatry (over 3 million views), and blogs entitled "In Defense of Anti-Psychiatry" hosted on websites such as "Mad in America." Comments left by viewers will read "psychiatrists are beyond brutal and have no conscience" and "the most we can hope for is that [psychiatrists] be exposed and brought to justice in our lifetime."

Online spaces that share differing perspectives about psychiatry can become unproductively heated. Some patients can feel that their lived experiences are invalidated, and some mental health professionals can feel attacked. The science, unfortunately, is often lost in disputes that elevate anecdotal evidence from all parties, resulting in a breeding ground for misinformation.

"Don't Wanna Be a Canadian Idiot"

You probably haven't heard of the Citizens Commission on Human Rights (CCHR), but if you walk down the street of Sunset Boulevard in Los Angeles, California, just a few blocks away from major LA landmarks, such as Amoeba Records and the Hollywood Palladium, you can gain free entry into one of its buildings, a multi-million-dollar museum. But it's no ordinary museum. Plastered on the outside above its entrance is an eye-catching white sign with bolded red and black font reading "Psychiatry: An Industry of Death." Inside, the building lights up with posters of terrified faces, tortured bodies, and Holocaust imagery. On opening night in 2005, it was reportedly attended by well-known celebrity members of the Church of Scientology, such as Catherine Bell, Jenna Elfman, Priscilla and Lisa Marie Presley, Danny Masterson, and former Scientologist Leah Remini.

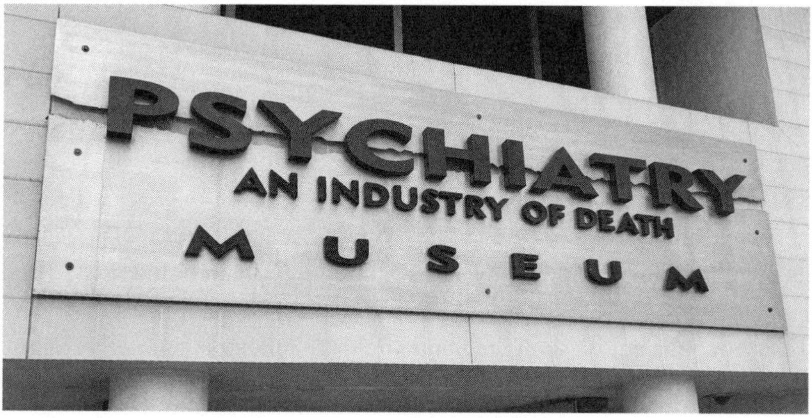

Not too long ago, the CCHR briefly made news headlines in Canada. I can recall watching with interest as students at the University of Ottawa bravely protested at their school. "Psychiatry: An Industry of Death" had gone mobile and set up shop as an exhibit on campus. In response, students gathered to fight against the exhibit's stigma toward psychiatric treatment. Some of their signs read "I've been on sertraline for 2 years come @ me," "Mental health services matter," "Science: check your facts, we need psychiatry," "Students need support not stigma," and "Don't wanna be a Canadian idiot." The University of Ottawa Student's Union and the university president,

Jacques Fremont, voiced solidarity. Fremont stated, "We support evidence-based science. We are with you."

So what's the CCHR? Some describe the organization as a front group for the Church of Scientology, while others say it's really an arm. The CCHR website admits that it was "co-founded in 1969 by the Church of Scientology and Professor of Psychiatry Emeritus Dr. Thomas Szasz." Yes, *that* Szasz. The website continues:

> CCHR functions solely as a mental health watchdog working alongside many medical professionals including doctors, scientists, nurses and those few psychiatrists who have taken a stance against the biological/drug model of "disease" that is continually promoted by the psychiatric/pharmaceutical industry as a way to sell drugs. . . . People frequently ask if CCHR is of the opinion that no one should ever take psychiatric drugs, but this website is not dedicated to opinion. It is dedicated to providing information that a multibillion dollar psycho/pharmaceutical industry does not want people to see or to know.

If that passage sounds fallacious and conspiratorial to you, that's because it is. The Church of Scientology was an integral part of the original anti-psychiatry movement. It's been waging a war on psychiatry since its inception, looking to eradicate psychiatric practice and replace it with its own brand of pseudoscience. Its founder, science fiction writer L. Ron Hubbard, wrote in 1969: "There is not one institutional psychiatrist alive who . . . could not be arraigned and convicted of extortion, mayhem and murder." That same year, Hubbard and Szasz founded the CCHR, which continues to disseminate anti-psychiatry propaganda to this day with its exhibits, widely available documentaries, and social media. According to their nonprofit publicly available tax documents, the CCHR spent more than $2.3 million in 2019 on "research," an "informational clearinghouse and hotline," "public education and advocacy," and "other program services."

While Scientologists can regularly be found protesting outside of psychiatric conferences and meetings, they are also busy promoting their own pseudoscientific approaches to mental health. For example, one approach called the Introspection Rundown—composed of solitary confinement, vitamins, calcium, and magnesium—was reportedly involved in the death of member Lisa McPherson in 1995, whereby Scientology was indicted on two felony charges related to abuse and neglect that were later dropped in a sea of controversy.

Scientology's drug treatment program, Narconon, has rehabilitation centers in more than 20 nations. If you go to their website, you will see pseudoscientific warning signs everywhere, such as the unethical use of testimonials and promotion of claims divorced from the broader scientific literature. For example, they promote a "drug free withdrawal" program, which is not recommended in the case of alcohol or opioid addiction because withdrawing from those substances can produce dangerous and life-threatening symptoms that are most effectively managed under medical supervision with the use of medications. You will also see a "new life detoxication" program that largely consists of having people ingest megadoses of vitamins while sitting in a sauna. The aim is to "actually sweat out the harmful toxins naturally." Aside from this statement committing an *appeal to nature* fallacy—that is, the false belief that what is natural is good—it also dupes readers by using the medically nonsensical and common wellness industry buzzword "toxins."

Fittingly, Narconon avoids assistance from bona fide mental health professionals. In her book *Troublemaker: Surviving Hollywood and Scientology*, actress Leah Remini notes that "any form of psychoanalysis or therapy is completely frowned upon by the church." With no input coming in from qualified mental health experts, it's unsurprising that Scientology contributes to mental health misinformation in our culture, especially when amplified by celebrities.

Modern anti-psychiatry is not a monolith, and Scientology is only one of its facets. But no matter the source, common themes emerge that are remarkably similar and harmful to patients.

Grasping at Strawmen

Almost a decade ago, if you had told Annie Hickox that she and her daughter, Jane, would be shamed and stigmatized for their lived experience with mental illness, she would've thought twice about sharing their stories. When Annie first started to write about Jane's depression, she almost abandoned the project entirely, frequently breaking down in tears as she relived the painful memories. It was Jane who wouldn't let Annie off the hook and encouraged her mother to continue.

As Annie describes it, she was cooking dinner one evening when she received an unusual phone call from Jane. After the initial "hello," Annie couldn't hear Jane's voice. She asked, "Are you okay?" After a broken pause, Jane replied, "Mum, I can't do anything." Annie's heart already ached with knowing what that meant. As Jane described how she felt, Annie recognized many depressive symptoms: pervasive sadness, lack of interest in pleasurable activities, appetite and sleep changes, and a bottomless sense of failure. Mother mode then kicked in and she became hellbent on finding Jane help.

As a teenager, Annie too had experienced depressive symptoms, including a prolonged period of emotional numbness. She says it's hard to articulate how it felt, paraphrasing the author Virginia Woolf, who stated: "When describing illness, language runs dry." But Annie does an impressive job nonetheless. She says, "In a very real sense I felt absolutely nothing, even about nothingness itself."

In her late teenage years, Annie also developed harrowing psychotic symptoms. She believed that she suffered from syphilis—despite having the sketchiest idea of the symptoms—and that she had long, maggot-like creatures embedded under her skin. She believed that her legs were slowly but visibly withering away, that her clothes could catch on fire from static electricity during her sleep, and that she could hear alien beings behind the closet door laughing because of how frightened she was that they were monitoring her thoughts and movements.

It hasn't been easy for Annie to share these very personal experiences, especially since, for over 35 years, she has been working in the United Kingdom as a clinical psychologist. She decided that even though she has felt intense shame, a sense of failure, and like an imposter in her workplace, it was vital to write about juggling her roles as mother, patient, and mental health professional. Her essays were featured by the British Psychological Society as well as on BBC Radio in London. This was Annie's and Jane's way to fulfill their goal of potentially helping even a single reader to feel less alone. "Mental health cannot enter the conversation if we don't let it in," Annie told me.

I have immense respect for Annie and Jane, not only because they've done their part to decrease stigma and improve mental health literacy, but also because they did it while withstanding acerbic attacks on their exposed vulnerability. I wouldn't blame them if they wanted to retract their pieces. In sharing their stories, Annie was overwhelmed by public support from patients and professionals alike who could relate to their emotional rollercoaster. But she was also met with stigma cloaked in misinformation.

On social media, it was suggested that she had "medicated her daughter" and was "unfit to work as a mental health professional" because she's "probably mentally ill" and "on drugs herself." Annie told me that the stigma was even more striking when these messages came from members of our own profession. A clinical psychologist described her article as evidence that she was "dragging" Jane into a self-serving drive to support diagnosis and psychiatry. In response to Annie taking Jane to see her family physician, a psychotherapist stated, "What a shame you went straight to a bio bio bio treatment without addressing the root causes."

Oozing from the vitriol directed toward Annie and Jane are anti-psychiatry sentiments. In the age of social media, these sentiments become amplified and far reaching. If you pay close attention to their content, stripped of the personal way they're conveyed, you'll notice themes beneath the attacks.

A trope is defined as a recurring, overused phrase, idea, or theme. Common tropes of anti-psychiatry continue to circulate each day in popular culture and social media—and even in academia—as if they are brand new and unrefuted. As I divulged in Chapter 2, these tropes show up at my hospital clinic and interfere with patient care. And as a seasoned veteran of X (formerly Twitter), I've seen too many online that often and unfortunately remain unchallenged.

In 2020, I decided that I'd seen enough. I tracked down and recruited two extraordinary psychiatrists, Joe Pierre and Tyler Black, to help me distill and highlight these tropes. Together, we published them in an online article. Since then, we've noticed even more pop up. I've included an updated, nonexhaustive list, along with our corrections, under the heading "Anti-Psychiatry Tropes and Corrections," on pages 199–200 in "Mind the Takeaways."

These tropes are sticky. They're like cockroaches of mental health misinformation: No matter how many times they're addressed and debunked, they just won't die. Like the nature of propaganda itself, their stickiness can be explained by the fact that they contain distorted kernels of truth. In other words, anti-psychiatry tropes take the form of strawmen fallacies, which are distortions of an argument that are weaker and easily defeated versions of the actual argument. Attacking a cartoon depiction of psychiatry by misrepresenting its positions as made of straw and devoid of nuance can be powerfully persuasive.

For example, at the opening of this chapter, we saw Tom Cruise proclaim that "there is no such thing as a chemical imbalance." Ironically, psychiatry would agree with him. The problem is that Cruise used that fact to argue that Brooke Shields shouldn't use antidepressant medications to treat her postpartum depression. That argument is a strawman fallacy.

The "chemical imbalance" trope is a myth that derives from the monoamine hypothesis of depression, which dates back to at least the 1950s. It predicted that the underlying pathophysiological basis of depression was a depletion in the levels of particular neurotransmitters in the central nervous system, such as serotonin, norepinephrine, and dopamine. Nowadays, this hypothesis is no longer taught. Scientific evidence has shown us that the way the brain interacts with antidepressant medications is vastly more complex than suggested by the oversimplified monoamine hypothesis. The current position of psychiatry is that antidepressant medications work but that we are still in the very early stages of understanding why they work and for whom.

Grasping at strawmen is an effective strategy if the aim is to demonize psychiatry. Tragically, it's a counterproductive strategy if the aim is to improve legitimate issues, such as patient autonomy, overdiagnosis, overprescribing practices, obtaining fully informed consent for medications, and the profit-driven influences of "Big Pharma" and insurance reimbursement. Like any health care profession, there will always be variability in terms of the quality and ethics of individual clinicians. It's disingenuous to use those differences in an attempt to discredit an entire scientific profession. Unethical and incompetent care are certainly the common enemies of psychiatry and anti-psychiatry.

Yet the extremism of modern anti-psychiatry overshadows its merit and generates a repository of misinformation. It stigmatizes and invalidates the lived experience of patients, like Annie and Jane, and the countless people who have benefited from evidence-based, psychiatric care. It attempts to rob people of the opportunity to seek such care. And it keeps me up at night because it negatively interferes with the recovery of my own patients and those who continue to reach out to me to share their stories. Ultimately, it's a pseudoscientific assault on public health.

* * *

The history of psychiatry is morbid. No question about it. It grew in parallel with the history of the anti-psychiatry movement and reflected the nascent science and cultural context of its time. All health professions must learn from their missteps and confront their pasts.

Today, psychiatry remains imperfect and must continue to evolve in response to scientific criticism. The science of psychopathology is messy because mental health and illness are messy. But just because they're messy doesn't mean we know nothing about them or how to help people. It doesn't mean that mental illness is a myth, that psychiatric medications are useless or more harmful than helpful, or that psychiatrists only care about pushing medications. It can be hard for the average person to sift through this misleading noise that appeals to our emotions and biases.

Still, there isn't an anti-cardiology movement. No one is protesting pediatricians or aggressively chanting outside of emergency medicine conferences. Psychiatry, as a medical specialty, and unlike clinical psychology and other allied mental health professions, is unique in its capacity to serve as a lightning rod for anti–medical establishment sentiments and in taking most of the heat for our gaps in knowledge about mental disorders and their treatment. And where there are gaps, there's exploitation.

The wellness industry and modern anti-psychiatry were destined to be bedfellows. Both exist as foils to the medical industry at large. When we peek behind the curtain, we discover that they share similar underlying pseudoscientific foundations, tactics, and tropes. Think: the chiropractor who denies the existence of mental illness but says they can "address the root cause" of your mental health concerns by charging you for a spinal adjustment; or the acupuncturist telling you their needles can unblock your chi without the side effects of psychiatric medications; or the integrative medicine practitioner who wishes to sell you a new diet and detox plan to rid your body of the "toxins" that are the real source of your troubles. Ultimately, the wellness industry capitalizes on our gaps in knowledge by filling them with pseudoscientific caulk. Let's get to know the history and ingredients of that caulk more in depth in the next couple of chapters.

4

The Wellness Industry

Alternative Medicine as the Perfect Con Game

When most people hear the name Kellogg, they think of breakfast cereal. Corn Flakes, Rice Krispies, maybe even Eggo Waffles and Pop-Tarts. Misogynistically removing the clitoris as a punishment, masked as a treatment for female sexual promiscuity and masturbation, is not top of mind. Yet these kinds of moralizing ideas about health—embraced and perpetuated by a health authority of Kellogg's significance—gave birth to the modern wellness industry and have become rooted in alternative medicine.

In 1878, John Harvey Kellogg and his brother, Will Keith, built something called the Battle Creek Sanitarium. It was once a world-famous medical center, spa, and grand hotel, attracting the wealthy and preeminent celebrities of its day. While Will helped run the sanitarium before starting the now multi-billion-dollar Kellogg cereal company, John went on to become one of America's most popular physicians and bestselling authors. The advice dispensed by John in his books, lectures, and *Good Health* magazine was followed by millions, and in 1921, his research on digestion and diet was nominated for a Nobel Prize.

But amid his brilliance was also folly. He was on a self-appointed, messiah-like mission from God to make the world healthier and was derided by colleagues for his grandiose personality. Many of his ideas blended medical concepts with Seventh-day Adventist Christian beliefs on health reform. The result was a philosophy that natural, wholesome living combined with faith in God made the best medicine.

The term *wellness* wasn't even around yet. Instead, to obtain the lifestyle he idealized, John prescribed the precursor to wellness—what he called *biologic living*. It meant striving for health in mind, body, and spirit to prevent illness, but doing so with three panaceas: physical exercise, adequate sleep, and a diet replete with fruits, grains, vegetables, and milk. Literally every health condition could be treated with that trifecta recipe.

He warned patients against sedentary lifestyles, meat, sugar, caffeine, tobacco, alcohol, sex, and obesity—the latter of which was considered both a slight against physical attractiveness and a health hazard. He referred to masturbation as "self-abuse," advising that it could lead to mental illness, cancer, and moral destitution. In boys, it was to be treated by circumcision if bandaging their hands didn't work; in girls, he recommended pure carbolic acid to the clitoris, as well as its removal along with the labia minora of the vulva.

According to medical historian Howard Markel, John was obsessed with cleanliness and virtuous eating. He believed that digestion could be aided by chewing food to oblivion and would guide his dinner guests in a round of the "Chewing Song," with the chorus beginning, "Chew, chew, chew, that is the thing to do." He also told his patients they should have four or five odorless bowel movements a day. Occasionally, he would leave social gatherings, only to return with a container of his most recent fecal specimen, and then place it under the noses of his friends to brag about its sweet and odorless quality.

Quirks aside, John was developing and promoting his ideas at the dawn of modern medicine in North America. Something called the Flexner Report of 1910 ushered in this era. The book-length report written by Abraham Flexner embraced rigorous science and its advancement as the new ethos of health care. Although the report raised the quality of medical education, it simultaneously hurt disadvantaged communities by shutting down rural and historically Black medical schools and revising entrance requirements to medical schools that worked against those who were economically underprivileged by making them more arduous and expensive. Schools that offered training in alternative medicine—such as naturopathy, homeopathy, and chiropractic—were told to drop it from their curriculum or shut down as well.

By the time John died in 1943, modern medicine was an entrenched scientific enterprise. But the aftermath of the Flexner Report left something to be desired. As Thomas Duffy, a professor at the Yale School of Medicine, put it, the hyperfocus on excellence in science was not well balanced by a comparable push for excellence in clinical care. In other words, some physicians became coldly distanced from patients in a way that allowed nurses and alternative medicine practitioners to step in and fulfill the warm art of listening, comforting, and humanizing.

In parallel with John's widespread promotion of biologic living, a man equally eccentric named Bernarr Macfadden was becoming the 20th century's first celebrity health influencer. He made millions selling Americans a bill of health that consisted of fitness, fasting as a cure-all, and hostility to medical science. Staunchly opposed to vaccination, he would strut around New York barefoot so his soles could absorb the Earth's energy, and he slept on the floor so his blood flow would align with its natural magnetic rhythm.

In 1899, Bernarr launched *Physical Culture* magazine, an assortment of articles about health advice alongside photos depicting scantily clad people (often him) showing off their physique. The magazine was a hit, leading to a New York–based publishing empire, and cementing Bernarr as an acclaimed health guru who sold the idea that "a person could exercise unqualified control over virtually all types of disease" given the willpower to live righteously.

I spoke with family physician and adjunct assistant professor Michelle Cohen, who has written about the legacies of John and Bernarr. "They were two of the most important health promoters of the 20th century and their influence continues into our time," she told me. "They brought 19th century ideas of health moralism into a new era of mass marketing and celebrity culture, championing the fantasy that your health could be controlled with a virtuous lifestyle."

Eating nutritiously and exercising regularly certainly matter for all aspects of health, including mental health and illness. But as Cohen brilliantly articulates, "There's a huge difference between lifestyle counselling and selling a cure-all based on lifestyle change. The former makes you a healthcare provider, the latter makes you a grifter."

Cohen also reminds us that "health is not a moral virtue." It's damaging when we hear disparaging comments about "lazy" people who "pop pills" and who use medication as a substitute for the hard work of eating "clean" and exercising.

These views especially apply to the nature and treatment of mental illness. Stigma festers and grows in the minds of those who unwittingly internalize the idea that mental illness is a sign of weakness or that taking medication is a personal failing.

The modern wellness industry inherited John's and Bernarr's moralizing attitudes toward health. Other historical and cultural threads too wove together to create the juggernaut of an industry that we see today. The fallout from the Flexner Report lingered into the advent of the counterculture movement of the 1960s and 1970s. These two social forces synergized anti–medical establishment societal attitudes that propelled patients into the welcoming hands of alternative medicine. Simultaneously, in late-20th-century North

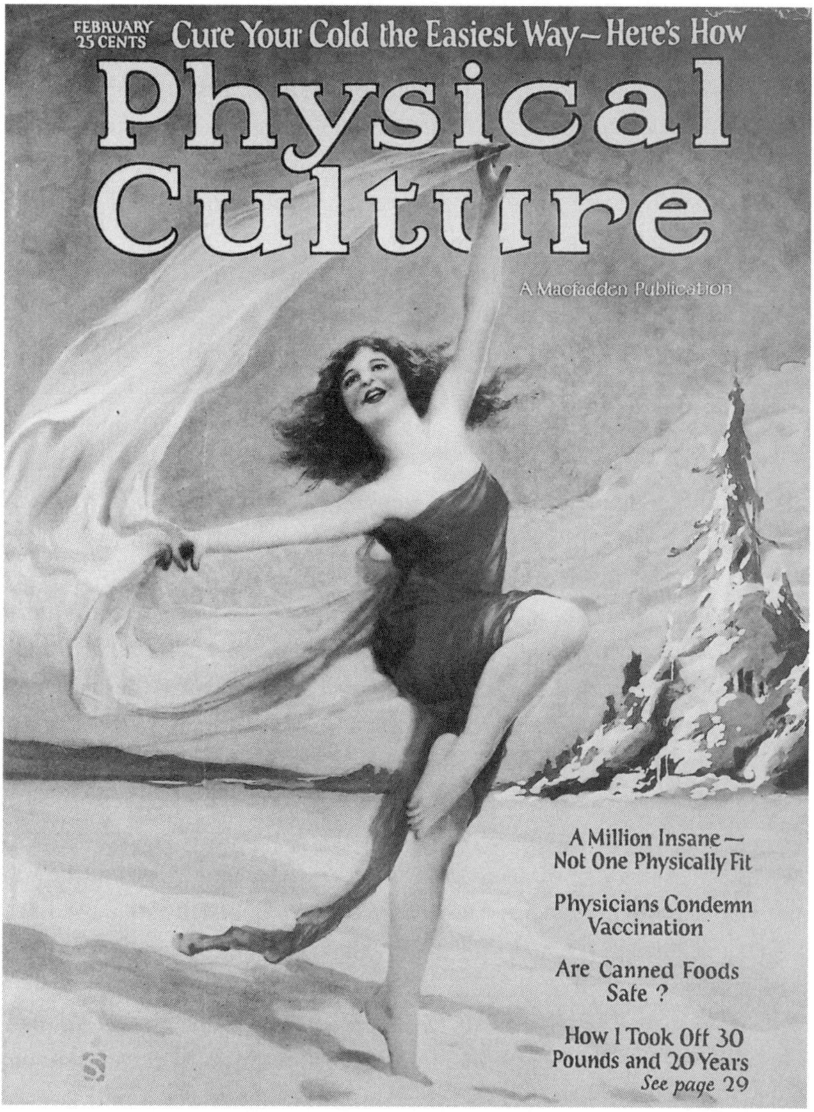

Source: *Physical Culture*, February 1924, Vol. 51, No. 2

America, people were increasingly identifying as consumers and demanding a wide range of choice whenever they spent money. This catalyzed a shopping cart approach to health care that magnified the role our own behaviors play in molding our health and led people to downplay the role of genetics and social factors, including plain old bad luck.

Sixteen years following John's death and 4 years after Bernarr's, the term *wellness*, as we use it today, was born. That's when the so-called father of the wellness movement, biostatistician Halbert L. Dunn, first used the term in the *Canadian Journal of Public Health*, in 1959. Reminiscent of the distinction described in Chapter 2 between mental illness and mental health, Dunn distinguished between good health—freedom from illness—and *high-level wellness*, defined as "an integrated method of functioning which is oriented toward maximizing the potential of which the individual is capable, within the environment where he is functioning."

Dunn's thoughtful definition didn't stick. "Wellness" quickly took on a life of its own.

Nowadays in many parts of North America, wellness has sprouted on every corner. Across from your local Starbucks, you'll see yoga and meditation classes interspersed with spa, weight loss, massage, acupuncture, and chiropractic clinics. Employee wellness programs offering subsidized gym memberships for work–life balance and mental health are a click away.

In her book *The Gospel of Wellness: Gyms, Gurus, and the False Promise of Self-Care*, journalist Rina Raphael laments how there's no agreed-upon definition of wellness, noting that it's one reason the industry has grown so big: "Wellness has devolved into an ambiguous marketing term that can just as easily mean activated charcoal toothpaste as it does mindfulness." It has seemingly ballooned to include anything and everything. Ask one guru what they mean by wellness and receive a different answer from the next.

Within its disorder, there's paradoxical order. In her analysis of the way that wellness promoters use the rhetorical power of language, associate professor Colleen Derkatch has caught the industry red-handed. In *Why Wellness Sells: Natural Health in a Pharmaceutical Culture*, she beams a light on two opposing messages that bombard marketing materials and drive sales: On the one hand, we're told that we need wellness to enhance, boost, and optimize our health; yet on the other, we're sold products and services designed to treat health conditions and restore what we're missing. We hear something like "maximize your mental health" by "treating your energy blockages and diet deficiencies." The term *wellness* has drifted from Dunn's definition and morphed into dollar signs, drawing us into a never-ending cycle of enhancing our health by treating problems we didn't know we had.

The wellness industry is currently valued at a breathtaking $5.6 trillion worldwide, which includes earnings from bona fide resources for healthier living (e.g., sports and exercise classes) as well as alternative medicine products and services. It also includes what's been dubbed the $181 billion global mental wellness economy, to capture money spent on sleep services and monitors, meditation and mindfulness resources, supplements for "brain health," cannabis and psychedelics, and self-help delivered by gurus, coaches, organizations, and apps.

Most perniciously, wellness has come to represent a wonderland free from the constraints of scientific scrutiny. The beating heart of the industry flows with pseudoscience, and to say that it's lucrative would be an understatement. It's the commercial home to the alternative medicine industry itself, estimated to be worth nearly $200 billion worldwide in 2025. In the United States alone, Americans spend over $30 billion per year on alternative medicine, and even the homeopathy industry is valued at $1.2 billion, used by an estimated 5 million adults and 1 million children.

Branding and Rebranding

As I've studied alternative medicine and its advertising in the mental health realm, I've found that it's as sly and adaptable as some of the charismatic grifters who read from its script. To be fair, not all promoters of alternative medicine are aware of what they're parroting. But repeat a lie often enough and it becomes your truth. Commodified alternative medicine is an ideology. It's not merely a set of unsupported and pseudoscientific health practices that prosper at the borders of evidence-based health care.

Baked into alternative medicine are moralizing attitudes handed down from the early evolution of the wellness industry. It has its own tropes (that we'll learn about in the next chapter) to propagate distrust in mainstream health care, and its own fallacies to cajole audiences (that we'll see in Chapter 6). It also shapeshifts in its name to sneak pseudoscience into the health care system at large.

Historically, alternative medicine has been called *drugless healing*, *fringe medicine*, *holistic medicine*, *irregular medicine*, *medical cultism*, *medical sectarianism*, *natural healing*, and *unconventional medicine*. The term *alternative medicine* began to be used in the 1970s. And according to medical historian James C. Whorton, it's loaded. The word "alternative" juxtaposed with "medicine" suggests that alternative medicine competes with mainstream medicine while simultaneously connoting a modicum of "medicine's" legitimacy. It implies somewhat of a false balance in two approaches to health, regardless of what the science has to say.

The rhetorical trickery continued as time went on. In the 1990s, the acronym *CAM* was coined to represent the term *complementary and alternative medicine*. In this sleight of hand, adding the word "complementary" conferred more legitimacy to alternative medicine by subtly transforming its image from a fishy, backup option to one that could be used alongside mainstream medicine. Shortly after, the term *integrative medicine* emerged, pioneered by Andrew Weil, a Harvard-trained physician and bestselling author, even further suggesting that alternative medicine could be "integrated" into the mainstream health care system. And then came *functional medicine*, a deceitfully vague term invented by Professor Jeffrey Bland to sell dietary supplements, and shot to fame by its poster boy, physician Mark Hyman, who became a medical advisor to Bill and Hillary Clinton.

Let me show you an example of the smoke and mirrors. One of Hyman's *New York Times* bestselling books is called *The UltraMind Solution: Fix Your Broken Brain by Healing Your Body First: The Simple Way to Defeat Depression, Overcome Anxiety, and Sharpen Your Mind.* Take note of the choice in language. The immediate message in the title is that if you experience depression or anxiety, your brain is *broken*, and Hyman can gift you a *simple way* to remedy your suffering. What's the remedy? When we open the book, we're introduced to this idea: "To achieve optimal health, your body needs to be balanced in the seven keys to UltraWellness. Balance in these seven key systems in your body, help your broken brain fix itself. This is the revolutionary truth that is the foundation of *The UltraMind Solution.*"

Except it's hardly revolutionary. It's the same moralizing alternative medicine grift that's been promoted since the time of John Kellogg and Bernarr Macfadden, consisting of Hyman's line of supplements to "maintain balance and enhance your brain chemistry" combined with diet and lifestyle change to "optimize your brain" and "live clean." A keen observer will also notice the mixed messages screaming from the pages—rhetoric that Derkatch has exposed as descriptive of how the wellness industry sucks us in with its linguistic gymnastics. That is, Hyman's protocol suggests that we can *enhance* and *optimize* by paradoxically *fixing* what's *broken*.

The imagery on the front cover of his book depicts a piece of broccoli protruding from an antidepressant pill bottle. It embodies an *appeal to nature* fallacy by hinting that a vegetable is an adequate replacement for medication. Dig into the book, and we're bombed with tropes derived from both anti-psychiatry (e.g., "These drugs [antidepressants] don't cure the problem. They cover over the symptoms") and alternative medicine (e.g., "If you have been diagnosed with 'mental disorders' or 'brain diseases,' I will tell you what you really need to know about the cause and cure for your suffering . . . as we understand the basic common molecular mechanisms at the root of your symptoms"). As the face of *functional medicine*, Hyman's jargon echoes the pseudoscientific, patient-blaming and pill-shaming rhetoric that has always defined alternative medicine propaganda. We just don't know if he's aware of the script.

The use of evolving, deceptive language in alternative medicine is also reflected in the branch of the U.S. government devoted to exploring its merit. The Office of Alternative Medicine was first established in 1991. It then became the National Center for Complementary and Alternative Medicine in 1998. When it transformed to its latest flavor in 2014, as the National Center for Complementary and Integrative Health, dropping the word "alternative," it was criticized for attempting continually to dodge the fact that it repeatedly and unethically funds scientifically implausible studies, such as investigating the effect of distant prayer in the treatment of AIDS and energy healing in the treatment of prostate cancer.

When I use social media to teach the perils of pseudoscience, one thing I notice is that many people are rightly confused about alternative medicine terminology. For example, when I explain that *integrative medicine* is just a fancy disguise for alternative medicine, people often ask me, "But isn't integrative care a good thing?" They're understandably perplexed about the word "integrative" because it's also used in health care settings to describe evidence-based collaboration on multidisciplinary teams among professionals. That kind of care isn't *integrative medicine*, but it's no accident that it sounds like it is.

Alternative medicine is a con game. Its various iterations—*CAM*, *integrative medicine*, and *functional medicine*—are marketing terms designed to confuse patients, promote pseudoscience, and sow distrust in mainstream medicine. And when these labels no longer serve as an adequate cover-up for pseudoscience, alternative medicine will be forced to rebrand once again.

Will That Be One Hat or Two?

Envision this scene: You're a licensed clinical psychologist working in a Canadian, publicly funded, hospital clinic. A patient has just walked into your office for their very first appointment. You're listening intently to their concerns, empathizing, validating, and doing your best to develop rapport. You're coexploring their mental life and it's starting to paint a picture of where to focus. They come back for a second session so that you can continue your assessment, this time with the use of semistructured diagnostic tools. They describe severe symptoms of anxiety to the point that they're incessantly worrying about everything from the future of their loved ones to poverty in developing nations to the traffic on the way home from the appointment. They tell you their worrying feels excessive, and they find it difficult to stop once they start. To help squash the anxiety, they've been using a benzodiazepine medication called lorazepam, multiple times per day, prescribed by their family physician. At this point, they crave the medication and feel like they've lost control over its use, which only makes the anxiety worse. Using the language of the *Diagnostic and Statistical Manual of Mental Disorders* to describe this aspect of their presentation, you think that they probably meet criteria for "generalized anxiety disorder" and a benzodiazepine addiction, captured by the category "sedative, hypnotic, or anxiolytic use disorder."

You decide it's time to talk about some treatment options. In a feat of magic, you've been given access to two hats. If you put on the first hat, you must proceed according to your licensing requirements and the codes of ethics laid out by the Canadian Psychological Association and the American Psychological Association. This means that you're obligated to provide evidence-based mental health care and cannot consider treatments that show no evidence of benefit and that may lead to harm, even if your patient consents. If you wear this hat, you and your patient would decide together on the best time to consult with a psychiatrist or physician with knowledge about how to initiate a slow, comfortable benzodiazepine taper to discontinue its use, and you would begin to discuss some psychotherapy options to target their anxiety, such as cognitive-behavioral therapy or psychodynamic therapy.

If instead you put on the second hat, you become liberated from the shackles of ethics. No longer burdened by the nagging of scientific evidence, you're free to offer any pseudoscientific treatment you wish. Homeopathy? Go for it. Energy medicine? Why not.

This scene is obviously preposterous. But it illustrates the very real ethical and legal dilemma faced every day by clinicians who offer alternative medicine. Timothy Caulfield coined its imaginary depiction of a choice between the two approaches as the *two-hats fallacy*.

The gist is this: Mental health professionals (and health care professionals more generally) cannot switch hats from being evidence based to not being evidence based, depending on the treatments they're offering. In other words, we can only wear one hat, and it's not the one adorned with pseudoscience. The ethical and legal reality creates an odd situation: If a mental health professional decides to offer an easily identifiable pseudoscientific treatment, such as Reiki, then they must tell patients that it doesn't work beyond the placebo effect and that there are other evidence-based treatments more likely to be effective.

Honesty is essential for a patient to provide informed consent. Clinicians who are not forthright about the relative benefits and risks of a treatment don't respect a patient's rights and individual choice. Where a cautionary yellow light is warranted for navigating the blurry clinical gray zone of new and promising treatments, a full-stop red light is the only response in the case of discredited pseudoscientific treatments. Here, science literacy matters: A choice between science and pseudoscience isn't a real choice, especially if you don't tell the patient which is which and if neither the clinician nor the patient can tell the difference.

Yet defiance of these ethical and legal requirements occurs all the time. A small research literature exists trying to estimate how often alternative medicine is used by people who experience mental health concerns, and it shows the rates are high around the world. For example, an American study found that 43% of people diagnosed with anxiety disorders reported using alternative medicine in the past 6 months, and a Swedish study of health care professionals working in psychiatric settings reported that 62% of them offered some form of alternative medicine. Another large study across 25 countries showed that alternative medicine use was 3.6% among people diagnosed with a mental disorder during the past year, and use was more common in high-income countries and among those who experienced greater severity of mental disorder symptoms.

Bottom line: People seek out alternative medicine.

In clinical practice, there are wins and losses—heavy, human ones. Battling alongside people every day who experience the confusion and ruin of severe mental illness and addiction is notoriously difficult. Sometimes, I receive emails from former patients updating me on their successes—and that's everything. Other times, I feel frustrated and helpless as I struggle to help people during the worst moments of their lives. Receiving news that a person has died is a dreadful inevitability, and words fail to capture the torment. So once again, I get people's desperation. I get why they turn to alternative medicine during times of vulnerability.

Still, pseudoscience under the guise of alternative medicine is no friend to patients. It's easy to trivialize alternative medicine as nothing more than harmless placebos. That's not what I'm demonstrating throughout this book, and it's not what the research quantifies. We know that Americans spend billions of dollars per year on dietary supplements despite extensive evidence that most are ineffective and sometimes harmful. More than 100,000 over-the-counter herbal and dietary supplements are available to purchase in retail stores and online in the United States, and they account for up to 20% of adult drug-induced liver injuries, which can lead to liver failure, requiring transplant. Various forms of vitamin supplementation have been linked to liver disease, pancreatitis, and thousands of visits to U.S. emergency departments every year, as well as increased risk of mortality compared to placebo. We know that alternative medicine of all forms can delay engagement with effective treatment, thereby potentially worsening symptoms on a patient's dime; that certain remedies interact badly with conventional medications; and that poor safety oversight in the herbal and dietary supplement market leads to higher risk for toxic contamination. Above all, the harms of alternative medicine need to be weighed against its practically nonexistent benefits.

One might protest and ask, "But if people want alternative medicine, then why can't you just give it to them? Why meddle? Who are you to decide what treatments they should have access to?" Fair enough. But the power that mental health care professionals possess is beholden to the deeply deliberated, historically rich literature on medical ethics that informs their license to practice. By that, I mean that their codes of ethics and legal standards of practice didn't just pop out of a vacuum, and they exist for good reason—in the service of people who are suffering.

When the Flexner Report of 1910 sounded the alarm for modern medicine to get its scientific act together and tighten the reins on what had been largely unscientific patient care, it inadvertently outsourced the art of healing. Alternative medicine had an eager ear to lend to patients who felt pushed away, and to this day patients find satisfaction in its presence. But it results in this sense of comfort not because homeopathy works or human energy fields are real, but because patients are soothed by feeling connected to practitioners who see and hear them—as well as factors that are common across all talk therapies that we'll learn about in Chapter 8.

In contrast to a strawman fallacy that portrays an argument in its weakest and most easily defeated terms, a *steelman argument* does the opposite: It gives credit where it's due by generously considering the strongest form of an argument. Steelmanning alternative medicine acknowledges its best features, which are its practitioners' ability to spend more time with patients and cultivate the power of a therapeutic relationship, which reveals itself as a secure emotional connection between patients and clinicians. The short 10-minute appointments with family doctors and the dangerously long wait times to see specialists in mainstream medicine just don't cut it.

This is a real problem—but it's a system one. When given the time, resources, and training, evidence-based health care professionals can provide the same art of healing that is capitalized on by alternative medicine practitioners, leaving the pseudoscience behind. And it just so happens that the art of healing is what mental health professionals are specifically trained to do—seeing and hearing patients is their forte. As the late physician and skeptic Harriet Hall has repeatedly said, "What alternative medicine practitioners do that is good is not special, and what they do that is special is not good."

Gaps in mental health care signal a call to fill those gaps with ethical, equitable, competent science and patient care. Gaps in mental health care don't justify filling those gaps with exploitation and pseudoscience masquerading under the banner of wellness and alternative medicine. Mental health care is only science informed and ethical if its clinicians are too. Declining to make a ton of money by selling and integrating alternative medicine treatments into your practice because you hold patient care to be a more worthy priority is one way of demonstrating that you're a responsible clinician. To promote and practice pseudoscience remains unethical by the most basic standards because it deceives patients and threatens their health. Alternative medicine embraces an approach to mental health care that abandons ethics and reduces the rigor and role of science in the alleviation of distress. That's not the hat that I chose, and it's not the one that will improve public health.

Blank Shingles

Choosing a career isn't an easy decision. Many people with kind hearts and caring souls are drawn to the helping professions because they wish to make a positive impact on the lives and health of others. Those who enter psychology, social work, nursing, medicine, and other allied health disciplines get that opportunity—but with the caveat that they use their license ethically and in accordance with the standards set by the regulatory organization that legally oversees their profession. For example, my own license to practice as a clinical psychologist is issued by the College of Alberta Psychologists. The title of "psychologist" is legally protected in many countries—it can't be used unless a person meets certain education and registration requirements. The reason that all regulatory bodies exist in the first place is to protect the public from harm and malpractice. In theory, we only get to wear one hat.

Once we open our favorite social media app, the landscape blows wide open. Virtual shingles are hung by some equally kind hearts and caring souls, but ones who are unlicensed. They go by any number of legally nonprotected titles, because there are no regulatory bodies overseeing their fields of practice. A "holistic mental wellness coach" can charge you for sessions to treat your depression without any training, and a random person from New York State can call themselves a "mental health clinician" on a whim. Many people are surprised to learn that, depending on the country or jurisdiction, other popular professional-sounding titles aren't protected either, such as "therapist," "psychotherapist," "counselor," and "practitioner." That means anyone can set up a business and legally market themselves on Instagram using those descriptors right now if they choose.

When people use unprotected titles to treat mental health and illness, they have free rein: They're obviating expertise, codes of ethics, legal standards of practice, and overall accountability to patient care. Doubly worse: They do so in the context of the wellness industry, which largely doesn't regulate its products and services. Say what you rightly will about the perils and history of corruption in the $1.4 trillion pharmaceutical industry, but unlike the wellness industry, at least Big Pharma aspires to be regulated for safety.

As a patient, when poop hits the fan, you want regulatory bodies in your corner. If you long to hire a "coach" for motivational purposes and to help you achieve your life goals, then that's wonderful, and all the power to you. Ethical problems start to emerge, however, when those "coaches" begin to offer mental health care services with no qualifications, such as the ability to assess and treat a person's addiction concerns, depression, anxiety, or trauma. One consequence of unlicensed practitioners in a largely unregulated wellness industry is that there's no recourse to file complaints and correct any wrongdoings. When treatment goes awry, there's not much you can do aside from sludging through the emotional and financial stress of filing a civil lawsuit.

In a twist of absurdity, some alternative medicine disciplines *are* regulated. For instance, naturopathy is regulated in five Canadian provinces, meaning that the titles of "naturopathic doctor" and "naturopath" are protected. Even the title of "homeopath" is protected in Ontario, the only province in Canada with a regulatory body that governs the practice of homeopathy. I didn't just use the word *absurdity* to be facetious. I meant it literally. Regulatory bodies that fail to protect the public undermine their own mandate—and that's precisely what alternative medicine regulatory bodies do by virtue of legitimizing and governing pseudoscientific disciplines.

The absurdity in Canada made headlines recently when a naturopath named Jason Klop petitioned the British Columbia Supreme Court. Klop was under investigation by the College of Naturopathic Physicians of British Columbia for treating autism by unsafely manufacturing and selling both pills and enemas made with his nephew's feces for approximately $15,000, even though it's an unproven treatment and could put children in danger. Klop's lawyer argued that the investigation was unnecessary because naturopaths are "not bound by science." "What does it take for a naturopath to do something so unbecoming in a field that is so broad and open to interpretation?" he posed to the court.

Even though his lawyer lost the case, he has a point. It's unclear what's worse: a grifter with no license and no accountability or one with a license and feigned accountability.

Ugly Marriages

It's undeniable that America has a gun violence problem. On December 14, 2012, Adam Lanza died by suicide after murdering 20 students and six staff members at Sandy Hook Elementary School. To add to the agony of an already despairing community, numerous conspiracy theories surfaced doubting what had transpired. The most popular one disputed that the massacre even occurred, with claims that it was an elaborately orchestrated hoax by the political left to advocate for stricter gun control. It was broadcasted by Alex Jones, a radio host for *The Alex Jones Show* and infamous conspiracy theorist. Parents of the children who died have been suing Jones and his company for several years, leading him to file for bankruptcy and owe billions of dollars in damages—but it hasn't been enough to shut down his operation.

When I went to Jones's website, InfoWars, I was immediately accosted by an advertisement: "Amp up your body's probiotic potential with prebiotic fiber—Back in Stock 40% off—Shop Now." Then I clicked on his InfoWars

Store and the "Health & Wellness" section, which took me to virtual shelves of more dietary supplements: "Better Mood +" for $59.99; "Mushroom Max Nootropic" for $59.99; "CBD Full Spectrum 1000 mg" for $89.99; "Immune Support" for $29.95; there was even an "Alex Jones Was Right—Fundraiser Shirt" for $24.95.

What is going on here? Why would a far-right conspiracy theorist be peddling wellness products that allege to provide "mood balance" and support your immune system "naturally with ultra-high qualities selected for their nature-based benefits"?

According to *New York Times* journalist Farhad Majoo, stoking conspiracy theories is just a marketing tool for Jones—one that attracts people to his website and bombards them with ads for snake oil. It's what allowed Jones to generate an average of $55 million in annual revenue from 2016 to 2019.

Jones is not alone in marrying wellness with conspiracies. In 2009, the term *conspirituality* was first used as the name of a Canadian hip-hop group who sang about exposing political cover-ups and spiritual teachings. The term then appeared academically in the *Journal of Contemporary Religion* in 2011, as Charlotte Ward and David Voas used it to describe "a rapidly growing web movement expressing an ideology fueled by political disillusionment and the popularity of alternative worldviews." Then the Covid-19 pandemic happened, and the movement exploded.

Conspirituality is what it sounds like: a melding of the words *conspiracy* and *spirituality*. It has come to represent misinformation derived from the intersection of far-right conspiracies and left-wing New Age beliefs that epitomize wellness and alternative medicine. It shows up on the Instagram reels of wellness influencers who post anti-vaccine propaganda and sell dietary supplements while promoting QAnon, a conspiracy theory that a behind-the-scenes cabal of Satan-worshipping child abusers in U.S. government positions of power are running the world.

Derek Beres is a journalist and lead author of *Conspirituality: How New Age Conspiracy Theories Became a Health Threat*. He and his coauthors—cult researcher Matthew Remski and philosophical skeptic Julian Walker—also cohost the *Conspirituality* podcast devoted to understanding the movement and how it attacks public health.

I spoke with Beres about how conspirituality has contributed to mental health misinformation. "For decades, I've heard seemingly benign sentiments in yoga studios and at wellness conferences, things like: 'You're your own best doctor,' 'nobody knows your body better than you,' and 'food is your best medicine,'" he told me. These sentiments aren't benign. At their base, they reflect the deep-seated distrust in modern medicine that has always characterized alternative medicine and the wellness industry.

During the pandemic, vaccine hesitancy toward Covid-19 vaccines turned to *all* vaccines, rallying the anti-vaccine movement, and leading to outbreaks of treatable diseases like measles, whooping cough, and polio. Anti-vaccine conspiracies have emboldened people to distrust and criticize absolutely everything produced by pharmaceutical companies, including psychiatric medications. While Big Pharma has a lot of real problems, it's also become a battle cry for conspirituality sympathizers. As Beres told me, "You have wellness influencers offering supplements, yoga courses, retreats, breathing workshops, and so much more to alleviate depression, while some are explicitly claiming that people don't need medications to treat their mental health condition and that they can try this untested herb instead."

He's right. It's not only the potential adverse effects of supplements that can be dangerous, but also what treatments people are avoiding due to their beliefs. Far-right conspiracies give people in the wellness community even more reasons to be suspicious of mainstream mental health care. And just like Jones's store at InfoWars, those conspiracies are used to market pseudoscience. "Watch what they say, then watch what they sell," Beres warned me.

The anti-vaccine movement has had an ongoing love affair with the wellness industry dating back to at least the time of Bernarr Macfadden (*have another look at the cover of the* Physical Culture *magazine from earlier in this chapter*). This tracks with current research. One recent survey showed that vaccination rates tend to be lower among alternative medicine practitioners (e.g., naturopaths, chiropractors) compared to evidence-based health professionals, and one study evaluated 330 naturopath clinic websites, finding that 40 included vaccine hesitancy discourse and 26 offered vaccine or flu shot alternatives. Other kinds of research have shown that people who hold anti-vaccine attitudes tend to score high on measures of belief in conspiracies and tend to prefer alternative medicine to mainstream medicine.

The psychology behind conspirituality becomes strangely unsurprising when we consider the underlying commonalities shared by those who believe in conspiracies and those who gravitate to alternative medicine. Belief in one type of pseudoscience or conspiracy tends to attract multiple types, a phenomenon known—unsavory as the term might be—as *crank magnetism*. Research paints a complex picture of who is susceptible to such misinformation. As we'll learn about in Chapter 6, many variables come together and interact that place people at risk, such as their tendency toward conspiracy mentality, how high they score on a particular personality trait known as openness to experience, their tendency to believe pseudo-profound bullshit statements, their reliance on an intuitive thinking style, their lack of intellectual humility, and their mistrust of institutions and health care providers. It's a messy and developing picture to be sure, but it's one that unites around a recognizable psychology and helps shed light on why conspirituality exists.

Wellness and alternative medicine are promiscuous. In conspirituality, they form an alliance with far-right conspiracies. They've always had a not-so-secret love affair with the anti-vaccine movement, and as we discussed in Chapter 3, they were destined to be bedfellows with the anti-psychiatry movement. The glue holding these ugly marriages together is distrust in modern medicine. The inescapable offspring are mental health misinformation and pseudoscience.

Stolen and Weaponized

Not all distrust in modern medicine and mental health care is misplaced. Quite the contrary. As we learned in Chapter 2, science literacy involves understanding that science is a fallible human enterprise. Though hardly the norm, corrupt research and conflicts of interests in Big Pharma do taint the integrity of the health care system. We need to cultivate a healthy balance between skepticism and trust in expertise to best inform our health decisions. This is more difficult for minorities and other underprivileged groups with a history of oppression who have too many reasons to distrust the systems that continue to hurt them.

For example, it's well known that racism negatively impacts mental health in at least two ways. First, at the personal level, research shows that when someone perceives they're racially discriminated against, they're more likely to experience mental health concerns such as depression, anxiety, posttraumatic stress disorder (PTSD), poor sleep, distress, low life satisfaction, and low self-esteem. Second, at the societal level, *structural racism*—that is, the totality of ways in which racial discrimination shows up in various systems (e.g., housing, education, employment, earnings, media, criminal justice, science, health care, etc.)—permeates our culture, often leading to poorer quality of mental health care. We know, for instance, that minority groups are often overrepresented in the populations of American inner cities, where they receive treatment from lower-quality facilities with fewer clinicians who have lower clinical and educational qualifications than those in other neighborhoods. Given such an uneven system and both historic and current discrimination, is it any wonder that research shows ethnic and racialized minority groups are, on average, less likely to seek and receive mental health care services? Such distrust in the mental health care system is deserved. And the wellness industry is no welcoming beacon of inclusivity either.

In her book *American Detox: The Myth of Wellness and How We Can Truly Heal*, Kerri Kelly reminds us, "Today's wellness industry draws a lineage from South Asian and Indigenous cultures, that are often a part of spiritual traditions that employ a holistic and collectivist approach to well-being. Yet these practices have been divorced from their original contexts, distorted, and commodified to accommodate racist capitalist culture."

Most people are on board with the fact that pseudoscience is harmful. Yet some become uncomfortable when pseudoscience is exposed and corrected when branded as wellness or alternative medicine with roots in global cultures. This discomfort has landed in my inbox: "Thank you for debunking pseudoscience, but what about respecting other people's cultures and other ways of knowing?" some have asked me. My replies echo Kelly's observation.

Evidence-based mental health care works in the service of patients. Its philosophy assumes that good science is the best way to determine which interventions, no matter their origins, are safe and effective. When people argue that certain alternative medicine practices—such as Ayurveda or traditional Chinese medicine—should get a pass from scientific scrutiny, they're committing a logical fallacy called *special pleading*. The argument is that some practices should be immune from scientific evaluation without adequately justifying what makes the exception special. Sometimes, *special pleading* piggybacks on the *science of the gaps* fallacy (i.e., "science doesn't know everything") and the *appeal to tradition* fallacy ("the practice has been used for thousands of years").

It would be a disservice to patients to ignore cultural knowledge. Instead, it's the task of evidence-based mental health care to respect, study, incorporate, and practice in culturally competent ways, which is currently an active and evolving field within the mental health professions. The term *cultural competency* refers to a set of characteristics that every clinician should have, such as being sensitive to how their personal values and biases may impact their therapeutic relationship with patients, striving for knowledge about the culture and worldview of their patients, and skillfully working with patients in a manner that's culturally relevant. Scientists around the world have also joined a growing movement to make mental health care services more culturally competent by gathering evidence about how to best adapt evidence-based treatments, with changes that could include prioritizing discussions of pertinent cultural issues in psychotherapy (e.g., talking about stressors related to discrimination), adjusting the style in which treatments are delivered (e.g., including storytelling and folktales to relay psychotherapeutic concepts), and matching patients with clinicians based on their culture, ethnicity, or language.

Many years ago I worked with an Indigenous woman who wanted help quitting her alcohol and crack cocaine use. She had a horrid history laden with repeated sexual abuse during her upbringing on a local reserve and in foster care, developing PTSD along the way. Despite her adversities, she carried herself with the kindest demeanor and left an indelible mark on my growth as a clinician. One of the strategies that she used to stay abstinent was smudging: a sacred act used in many Indigenous rituals. It involves the burning of herbs—such as sweetgrass, sage, cedar, and tobacco—and then fanning the smoke to spiritually "cleanse" and "purify." When I asked her how she found it helpful, she explained that smudging made her feel more in touch with her identity and a sense of belonging to her community. Crucially, she refused to smudge while intoxicated out of respect to her Elders and community members, believing that it would be sacrilegious. We used her conviction to our advantage. Alongside her psychotherapy work, we ramped up the frequency of her smudging outside of sessions to strengthen her commitment to abstinence and planned other activities that increased her engagement in the community. We made it a point to discuss the traditional wisdom that she was connecting to her recovery, and she voiced pleasure in enlightening me about the teachings. As a young, fresh, non-Indigenous male clinician who felt out of his depth when it came to knowing how most helpfully to engage with her spirituality and cultural values, she was the first patient to really teach me what it meant in a practical sense to lean into cultural competency by embracing my own humility as part of this engagement and using our therapeutic relationship to guide aspects of treatment.

Cultural competency is written into the codes of ethics of the mental health professions such that every clinician needs to be dialed into its value. The wellness industry and alternative medicine do no such thing. They sell distrust in modern medicine. They frame their own practices as "exotic" or "ancient," but many of the most popular ones were developed relatively recently (see the next chapter). We're told that some practices emerge from "a different way of knowing," but then they're advertised using a scientific lens with claims that "it works" minus the evidential backing. Some authors have argued that practices such as Ayurveda and yoga have been culturally misappropriated and misused for profit, reflecting a phenomenon called Orientalism, which means cherry-picking, stereotyping, and romanticizing aspects of the Eastern world. If you have doubts, look no further than the "3-Day Ayurvedic Cleanse to Reset Each Season" meal plan advertised on Gwyneth Paltrow's Goop website, or to Kourtney Kardashian's "Go-To Ayurvedic Asparagus Soup Recipe" listed on her Poosh website.

Scientists and mental health professionals have plenty of work to do to win the trust of those who've been marginalized by our systems—but unlike grifters in the wellness and alternative medicine industries, at least they aren't selling back a culturally misappropriated bill of pseudoscientific goods.

* * *

The wellness industry owes a great debt to its forefathers. Celebrity doctors and wellness influencers of today resemble modern-era John Kelloggs and Bernarr Macfaddens, reincarnating many of the same tropes that moralize our mental health and berate mainstream medicine. Undue blame is laid at our feet if we don't eat right, feel right, or live medication-free.

Alternative medicine earns billions of dollars by scamming millions of people. It wears many masks, such as *CAM*, *integrative medicine*, and *functional medicine*, but no amount of finagling definitions can change the fact that pseudoscience is a built-in feature, not a bug of its foundations. Mental health professionals who embrace alternative medicine do so at the peril of patients and in contradiction to their ethical codes and legal standards of practice. It's a pernicious mistake to conflate wellness and alternative medicine with cultural competency. The former are retail outlets for pseudoscience, whereas the latter seeks to improve evidence-based mental health care by keying it into cultural frameworks without the pollution of grift.

Regulating health professions is supposed to protect the public, but it often fails, and is counterbalanced by unlicensed practitioners who can call themselves whatever unprotected title they wish as they sell services for any health condition they wish. Both misplaced and well-earned distrust in modern medicine contribute to mental health misinformation and sustain the wellness market. People are willing to turn a blind eye to the pitfalls of alternative medicine in part because it offers the warmth and human comfort that they may not be getting from the health care system.

As personalized and attentive as alternative medicine might seem, the mechanics are faulty. The term *lemon* is used to describe a newly purchased car that turns out to be defective: It may look pretty and might even get you to your destination a few times, but it has manufacturing issues and malfunctions that make it unsafe to drive. Alternative medicine is a lemon composed of pseudoscientific parts that jeopardize your mental health.

Let's now look under the hood.

PART 2

THE SIGNS TO LOOK FOR

5

Canaries in the Coal Mine

Warning Signs, Tropes, and Tactics

When he was 4 years old, Anthony William Coviello woke up one Sunday morning to an elderly man's voice speaking into his right ear. The man said, "I am the Spirit of the Most High. There is no spirit above me but God." Confused and alarmed when he saw no one in his room, Anthony ignored the voice but felt throughout the day like he was being watched. In the evening, at suppertime, he saw a "strange man" standing behind his grandmother at the dinner table with "gray hair and a gray beard" who was "wearing a brown robe." Anthony's family members didn't notice the man. He instructed Anthony to walk over to his grandmother and guided his hand to her chest. He then told Anthony to announce that his grandmother had lung cancer. In *Medical Medium: Secrets Behind Chronic and Mystery Illness and How to Finally Heal*, Anthony continues to tell us that he has been greeted by the man's voice every morning from that day forward as he's provided with paranormal information about the health status and necessary treatment of anyone he encounters.

Present day, Anthony is known professionally as the Medical Medium. On his website, you won't find a more impressive laundry list of praise for his healing abilities from celebrity stars and athletes, including Dwayne "The Rock" Johnson, Sylvester Stallone, Adam Sandler, Diane von Furstenberg, Robert De Niro, Hilary Swank, Gwyneth Paltrow, Novak Djokovic, Liv Tyler, Rashida Jones, Corey Feldman, James Van Der Beek, Naomi Campbell, Calvin Harris, and Courteney Cox, along with literally 50 other testimonials.

Anthony has been consulted by Kim Kardashian on her award-winning reality television series *Keeping Up with the Kardashians.* He has over 3 million followers on Facebook and over 4 million on Instagram. He is a *New York Times* bestselling author, publishing eight books about healing from health conditions, claiming on his website that his "unprecedented accuracy and success rate have earned him the trust and love of millions worldwide." His newest book, *Medical Medium Brain Saver*, purports to provide answers to "brain inflammation, mental health, OCD, brain fog, neurological symptoms, addiction, anxiety, depression, heavy metals, and Epstein-Barr virus."

In his books, blogs, and social media content, he outlines the causes and treatment of a vast array of health ailments, including mental disorders. According to Anthony, bipolar disorder, for example, has absolutely nothing to do with genetics but rather is caused by heavy metals in your brain—such as copper, mercury, lead, and aluminum—that can be inherited from your parents. The solution to bipolar disorder is to buy his books so that you can "detox" from these metals with a protocol of "healing foods" (i.e., cilantro, Atlantic dulse, spirulina, barley grass juice powder, and wild blueberries) and supplements (i.e., B_{12}, B complex, methylfolate, magnesium L-threonate, 5-HTP, California poppy, Micro-C, and zinc sulfate).

As you might have guessed, Anthony's assertions are false. They're not even close to being accurate. The scientific literature has shown that bipolar disorder has a huge genetic contribution. Some research has estimated that first-degree relatives of people who experience bipolar disorder have a nine-fold greater risk of developing the disorder than the general population. Bipolar disorder—like all mental disorders—is caused by a combination of genetic and environmental factors. It's not caused by a single gene, but rather its genetic contribution can be best understood as a combined effect across numerous possible genes.

You also won't find any legitimate research into people experiencing relief from bipolar disorder by "detoxing" from heavy metals. That science doesn't exist. Anthony, however, must know it doesn't exist and doesn't seem concerned, because as noted on his website he is provided with "extraordinarily advanced healing medical information that's far ahead of its time." On his blog, he states:

> There is a great deal of misinformation out there that can lead you to try something which doesn't actually work. This detox, the Medical Medium heavy metal detox, does work. . . . Research and medicine stay away from the discussion on toxic heavy metals. There is little to no conversation about them in medical communities, let alone in relation to how they cause mental disorders. There is so much controversy surrounding heavy metals that scientists do their best to neglect them altogether. As a result, medical communities are completely unaware of just how many illnesses toxic heavy metals play a role in.

By evading scrutiny from the scientific community and suggesting that scientists purposely neglect the relationship between bipolar disorder and heavy metals, Anthony is able to position himself as a health authority. To be fair, he does admit on his website that he's not licensed as a physician or any kind of health professional. But he also describes himself as a "chronic illness expert." Unlike other mediums, he doesn't merely claim to relay paranormal information about your deceased loved ones—rather, he's making bold claims about how serious health conditions are caused and best treated. Your ears should be splitting from the pseudoscientific alarm bells that are littered throughout his material. My intention in this chapter is to help you hear and spot such pseudoscience in the wild with your own senses. As misinformation-slaying author and gynecologist Jennifer Gunter once lamented with respect to Anthony's claims: "Is this what America really wants? Bad secondhand health advice from a ghost?"

Thinking Pseudoscientifically

In the late 1980s, some mental health researchers began to voice their concern that the dominant professional organization for psychologists in the United States, the American Psychological Association, was not focused enough on science. Chief among them was Scott O. Lilienfeld, who told the *New York Times* in 2004 that "many practitioners, because they don't keep up with the scientific literature, may be using suboptimal and, in some cases, even dangerous treatments." In 2020, Lilienfeld passed away too soon at the age of 59 amid devoting much of his career to teaching and exposing the many faces of pseudoscience in psychology and beyond. One of my biggest professional regrets is that I never reached out to him to express my gratitude for his brilliance and influence. He was survived by his wife, Candice Basterfield, who told me that he wished to persuade at least some of his colleagues that scientific thinking is an essential component of teaching psychology. His ideas need to be further popularized, especially in an increasingly digital age where the promotion of pseudoscience has grown and taken root in our culture.

We learned in Chapter 1 that there is no single criterion that draws a clear dividing line between science and pseudoscience. That would be too simplistic. Just as science is a complex, multifaceted construct, so too is its mimicry by pseudoscience. I've often pictured pseudoscience as a child that dresses as science for Halloween: It can thrive on magical thinking; it wants to trick you or take your resources; and if you squint, it sort of looks like science. While Lilienfeld and his colleagues likened the distinction between science and pseudoscience to the fuzzy boundary between day and night, the social psychologist Carol Tavris put it a bit more crudely when she once said: "Pseudoscience is like pornography; we can't define it, but we know it when we see it."

While that might sound facetious, it speaks to the fact that pseudoscience can be meaningfully differentiated even though its precise boundaries are unclear. Recall that pseudoscience is best identified by a constellation of warning signs, such that science differs from pseudoscience in degree rather than in kind. Determining pseudoscience is a probabilistic endeavor: The more warning signs that you hear and see, the greater the likelihood that you've unearthed something pseudoscientific. Get to know these signs. Memorize them if you can. To strengthen our grift detectors, we need to learn the following features of pseudoscience. (You can find an abbreviated list under the heading "Nine Red Flags of Pseudoscience" on pages 200–201 in "Mind the Takeaways.")

Nine Red Flags

1. ***Overuse of ad hoc hypotheses.*** An ad hoc hypothesis is a hypothesis that is added to a theory to save it from being proved wrong. It basically means introducing a new idea to explain away negative findings. For example, in the opening section of this chapter, when the Medical Medium stated that "research and medicine stay away from the discussion on toxic heavy metals," he was invoking an ad hoc hypothesis to make his claims about bipolar disorder immune from falsification.

   Another more formalized example is the essence of a 2018 essay called "Repositioning Individualized Homeopathy as a Psychotherapeutic Technique With Resolvable Ethical Dilemmas" that was published in the *Journal of Evidence-Based Integrative Medicine*—a pseudoscientific journal (we will learn about these kinds of journals later in this chapter). The essay's argument? Homeopathy doesn't work, but it can be kept alive if we call it a psychotherapy instead of a pharmacological intervention.

Scientists don't like seeing the use of too many ad hoc hypotheses, especially when they're used as loopholes to prevent refutation of a theory rather than improve upon a theory. Overuse of ad hoc hypotheses is a slimy tactic when used to justify claims that are clearly baseless.

2. ***Absence of self-correction.*** No scientific theory is perfect. In fact, most contain gaps in knowledge and have made predictions that turned out to be false. Whereas scientific theories can advance and evolve over time by learning from their errors, pseudoscientific theories remain stuck, stagnant, and stubborn. They don't move or improve. A classic example is astrology. Despite being around for the past 2,500 years and decades of research showing that it has colossally failed in every respect related to its theory and predictions of human behavior, your weekly Sunday horoscopes have barely changed from those of your distant ancestors.

   Another illustrative example is homeopathy. It has changed very little since it was born in Germany more than 200 years ago. Despite advances in the field of pharmacology, homeopathy is still partly based on the "law of minimum dose," which means the lower the dose of the medication, the greater its effectiveness. That baffling law might sound like it governs how molecules work in a parallel universe, and it's long been homeopathy's kryptonite. In the homeopathic world, less is more, where remedies typically are prepared by repeatedly shaking and diluting a substance—often, in water or alcohol—to such an extent that not a single molecule remains in the solution. Instead, homeopaths claim that a "memory" of the substance is left over that cures by activating the body's "vital force." The way that modern chemistry describes how molecules interact is at odds with these homeopathic ideas. Consider the implications too: If water had the ability to remember every substance it encountered, what a story it could tell.

3. ***Evasion of peer review.*** Science is a self-criticizing machine. One way that this occurs is by peer review, which essentially involves having experts in a scientific field grade each other's work and decide if it passes or fails. If you wanted to publish a study in a scientific journal, you would have to subject your study to the dragon's den or shark tank, so to speak, whereby experts would critically analyze and decide if your study is worthy of publication. People who promote pseudoscience are

experts at dodging the peer review process. They will either avoid it entirely or self-publish on blogs or websites or newsletters or social media. They will claim that their pet theories cannot adequately be tested with current scientific methods, or they will claim that the "scientific establishment" is biased against them. When the Medical Medium claimed on his blog that "there is little to no conversation about [heavy metals] in medical communities, let alone in relation to how they cause mental disorders," he was essentially evading peer review.

More cunning and insidious proponents of pseudoscience, however, will hijack the peer review system. They will publish their research and opinions in pseudoscientific journals among other like-minded pseudoscience fans, as was the case with the homeopathy essay above. Even scientific trash can be viewed positively by peers if they're partial to perceive it as pseudoscientific gold.

4. ***Emphasis on confirmation rather than refutation.*** Scientists are constantly and consistently trying to prove themselves wrong, whereas those who practice pseudoscience are more concerned with proving themselves right. The philosopher of science Imre Lakatos captured the spirit of this sentiment when he wrote that "the hallmark of scientific behavior is a certain skepticism even towards one's most cherished theories."

5. ***Reversed burden of proof.*** A classic indicator of pseudoscience appears when proponents reverse the burden of proof on skeptics to prove them wrong rather than having to provide evidence to support their own claims. The author Christopher Hitchens developed a philosophical rule—called Hitchens's razor—for what to do when it's encountered. He stated: "What can be asserted without evidence can also be dismissed without evidence."

6. ***Absence of connectivity to the broader scientific literature.*** This warning sign refers to theories lacking connectivity to other areas of scientific knowledge. It means that these theories are scientifically implausible because the principles that underpin them are completely divorced from the broader scientific literature.

   For example, as we've seen in the case of homeopathy, the "law of minimum dose" violates fundamental principles in pharmacology. Another textbook example is energy medicine. It's among the most confused and griftiest pseudoscientific approaches in alternative medicine because it purports the existence of a kind of human energy field that can be manipulated by energy healing practices, such as Reiki. If this were true, it would knock the bottom out of the entire field of physics. No such energy field has ever been found to exist, and its discovery would spark an existential crisis in every university physics department worldwide.

The Achilles heel of many unequivocal pseudosciences lies in their glaring scientific implausibility. For this reason, of all the pseudoscientific warning signs, this one perhaps carries the most weight.

7. ***Elevation of anecdotal evidence.*** We learned in Chapter 2 that the plural of anecdote is indeed not data, but misinformation. It doesn't matter if over 50 movie stars and celebrity athletes say that Medical Medium's healing protocols work. More reliable, higher-quality scientific data are needed to confidently make claims about the benefits (and harms) of treatments. No matter how many anecdotes you can accumulate, it will never be enough to show that a treatment works.

   Promoters of pseudoscience will elevate anecdotal evidence to sell their products and services. Recall that the use of patient testimonials—which are anecdotes—by psychologists in marketing materials and on websites is considered unethical, in part because it can result in inaccurate advertising. You won't find negative testimonials posted on the websites of those interested in selling pseudoscience; only the cherry-picked alleged hits matter, not the misses. Misusing anecdotal evidence is the currency of alternative medicine. It's endemic in the wellness industry and capitalizes on our susceptibility to falling for the *post hoc, ergo propter hoc* fallacy, resulting in powerful illusions of causality that can trick us into believing that a particular treatment works. Testimonials splattered all over a mental health professional's website are among the brightest of red flags. Ruthless adherence to anecdotal evidence in support of debunked pseudoscientific claims is a clue that ideology has punted critical thinking from the driver's seat.

8. ***Use of science-y sounding language.*** This warning sign is all about linguistic hocus pocus. It involves recruiting science-y sounding language to confuse and deceive people to legitimize research or sell products and services. An example might be the self-styled wellness guru who

speaks about "cells having the vibration of love" or claims that "each cell of the body contains 6 gigabytes of memory storing all physical and spiritual traumas." Ultimately, it's just bibble-babble, an inaccurate façade.

9. ***Absence of boundary conditions.*** Experts know what they don't know. Fake experts don't even know what they think they know. Scientifically plausible theories and treatments will state the conditions under which they do and do not apply. For example, chemotherapy will not be able to treat your depression. Pseudoscience, on the other hand, typically makes no such boundaries known. Instead, the floodgates open to an endless litany of conditions to which the pseudoscience can apply. Beware of people who profess to be able to treat almost any health condition, from mental disorders and back problems to indigestion and your cat's anxiety.

Pseudoscience as a Human Endeavor

Understanding the nature of pseudoscience involves more than just being able to identify its red flags. We also need to take the psychological and social context into consideration. Like science, pseudoscience doesn't happen in a vacuum but rather emerges from the fallible hands and minds of people who live in particular historical and cultural environments.

It's incorrect to plaster the label of pseudoscience willy-nilly from the privilege of a modern lens. For example, with 20/20 hindsight, it's easy to regard the ancient practice of trephination—a surgical intervention in which a hole is drilled into the skull—as a barbarically pseudoscientific way to release the evil spirits of those considered to be behaving abnormally. But within the context of their time and spiritual worldview, practitioners were sincerely making use of the best tools available to them. They weren't ignoring the broader scientific literature, evading peer review, or reversing the burden of proof. There were no viable alternative explanations to compete with their existing theories.

Scientific claims cannot be considered pseudoscientific merely by virtue of being debunked. Just as we dismiss trephination today, 200 years from now many of our current theories and treatments will appear scientifically implausible. Pseudoscience needs to be understood in light of the scientific advancements and sophistication of its time.

The Russian novelist Aleksandr Solzhenitsyn powerfully voiced that "the line dividing good and evil cuts through the heart of every human being." This idea means that we each have the capacity to act in ways that can tilt the world toward becoming a better or worse place. Solzhenitsyn's remark also applies to scientists. As we learned in Chapter 2, conducting science is not a neutral activity, but a human one. There are right ways to do science and there are wrong ways. Pseudoscience is the worst way.

It's devious. It's fake. It's derived from various combinations of science illiteracy, overcommitment to particular ideas, and in some, but not all, cases, malicious intent. The late Canadian psychologist Barry L. Beyerstein astutely noted that "even if promoters of pseudoscience are not intentionally trying to con you, it's entirely possible that they have conned themselves." It's perhaps those who have conned themselves who are the most dangerous, as they seek to con others in the name of ideological zealotry and misguided compassion. Personally, I would like to believe that grifters who are married to pseudoscientific beliefs are more influenced by poor science literacy than moral bankruptcy. Regardless, the underlying motivation is in some ways moot, because the end result is the same: No matter the intention, the act of conducting pseudoscience, particularly in the realm of mental health care, doesn't help anyone and most often makes things worse.

When teaching about pseudoscience to his students, Lilienfeld believed it was crucial to remain sensitive to these contextual nuances. I've summarized three of his tips below that we need to remember when scanning our surroundings for potential red flags:

1. ***Skepticism versus cynicism.*** The right attitude of a scientist is to be skeptical—not cynical—of claims and to question everything. A rookie mistake among those looking to question pseudoscience is to dismiss outlandish claims based on how absurd they sound rather than on evidence. If we chastise claims before we even entertain them, then we're acting in no better faith than the pseudoscientists who advance them. Simultaneously, skepticism is a tightrope, a balancing act. We don't want our mind to remain so open that grifters can easily fill it with fluff.

2. ***Scientific skepticism versus philosophical skepticism.*** This point is a bit tricky, but please bear with me. There's a difference between trying to understand reality with the scientific method (scientific skepticism) versus denying the idea that reality can be understood using the

scientific method (philosophical skepticism). Scientific skepticism is a good thing. It means understanding that scientific knowledge evolves over time and that some scientific theories have more evidence behind them than others. Philosophical skepticism, however, comes from a certain kind of philosophy called postmodernism, which can be used to undermine scientific truths. It essentially values subjective truths over objective truths and basically asks: "If all truths are equal, then who cares what science has to say?"

This kind of philosophical skepticism can provide a useful scapegoat for fans of pseudoscience because it allows them to dismiss scientific claims by saying something like, "Well, science can't know everything anyway!" This cop-out is slightly different than the science-of-the-gaps fallacy (to be discussed in Chapter 6), which sounds more like "Well, science doesn't have all of the answers." The difference is that those who commit the science-of-the-gaps fallacy are still acknowledging that science can provide an answer but contend that it just hasn't done so yet.

3. ***Pseudoscience versus metaphysics.*** Whereas pseudoscientific claims can be implausible, they can still be tested and lie inside the bounds of science. This differs from metaphysical and certain religious claims, which cannot be examined from a scientific perspective. For example, emotional freedom technique (EFT) is a pseudoscientific treatment for mental disorders based on the idea that your "energy field" can be manipulated and "balanced" by physically tapping certain points on your body. While implausible, the existence of "energy fields" and the procedure of tapping itself can be scientifically evaluated. This is unlike metaphysical claims, such as "God exists" or "an afterlife exists," which do not lend themselves to scientific scrutiny. That said, certain pseudoscientific claims made in the name of religion can indeed be scientifically debunked—for example, the creationist claim that Earth is only a few thousand years old.

Enter Alternative Medicine

It's the 10th week of your first science class in college and your instructor has given you an assignment. You're told you've been hired by the Mental Wealth

Company to create a social media advertisement for one of their latest products: either a diet detoxification protocol, a mental health–enhancing supplement, or a brand-new psychotherapeutic technique designed to treat mental disorders. The assignment is called "How to Sell Pseudoscience." After learning about pseudoscientific red flags earlier in the semester, you now need to weaponize and wield your skills by generating a catchy name and marketing your mental health product.

I would've loved to take this class during my undergraduate days. Students currently enrolled at Massasoit Community College in Massachusetts get that luxury. Melanie Trecek-King, an associate professor of biology, designed such a course from scratch. For more than a decade, she taught Introduction to Biology, a general education science class, to students who weren't aspiring scientists but rather needed to satisfy their science elective. In her experience, students took the class only because they *had to*, and they often ended the semester memorizing facts they'd soon forget and hating science just as much as or more than when they started. So in 2018, she scrapped that class and instead developed one focused on teaching critical thinking and science literacy. She figured that since we live in a society based on science, we need our citizens to be scientifically literate.

It paid off. Students now come to her class holding a variety of misconceptions but leave with their minds changed. She starts with teaching examples of pseudoscience and outright science denial that are less threatening to students' important beliefs or identity, such as witchcraft. "Since most students don't believe in witchcraft, they aren't emotionally triggered and can better explore the evidence," she told me. Throughout the semester, she slowly introduces other pseudoscientific claims involving ghosts, astrology, climate change denial, and alternative medicine. Exploring a range of topics better positions students to objectively evaluate their own views with varying emotional intensity.

The research literature, containing the work of Lilienfeld and colleagues, supports Trecek-King's approach. It shows that presenting and dispelling misconceptions in the classroom is an effective means of countering nonscientific and pseudoscientific beliefs. This jibes with Trecek-King's observation that "it's incredibly rewarding to watch students let go of long-held beliefs and realize they've been fooled: either by themselves or by charlatans."

Learning how to become a pseudoscientist can hopefully help prevent becoming one. The aim of Trecek-King's "How to Sell Pseudoscience" assignment is certainly not to train an army of grifters. It's to help open eyes to the

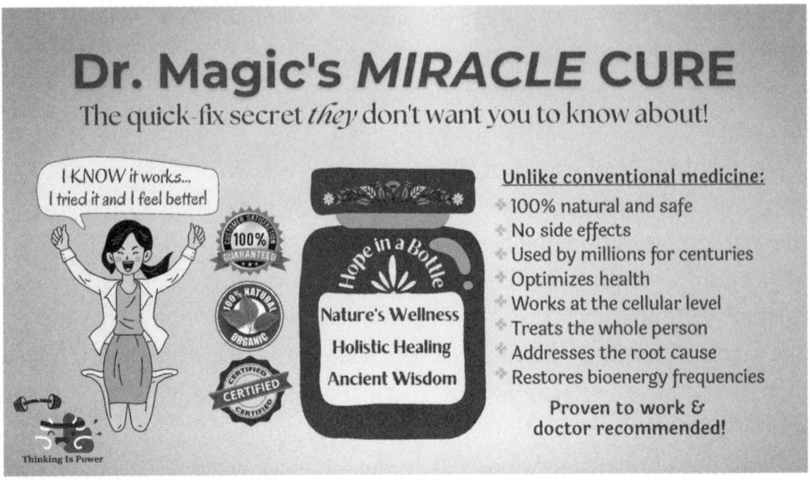

A fake advertisement for a generic health pseudoscience product created by Melanie Trecek-King. Can you spot the pseudoscientific red flags and alternative medicine tropes?
© Trecek-King, M. (2022)

workings of how alternative medicine is sold in the wellness industry. As one student said after their assignment, "Once you can see the techniques used to mislead people, they're very hard to unsee."

For over 30 years, Edzard Ernst has also been helping people to learn the trappings of alternative medicine. He became recognized as one of the world's foremost experts on alternative medicine by immersing himself in its culture as a patient, clinician, and scientist. According to a recent analysis, he was ranked as the most-cited researcher in the category of "Complementary & Alternative Medicine," which largely began in 1993 when he was appointed chair of complementary medicine at the University of Exeter, tasked with scientifically investigating all aspects of alternative medicine.

In numerous publications spanning decades, Ernst has contributed to detailing the ways in which those selling alternative medicine mislead people. For example, alternative medicine practitioners love to claim that in contrast to mainstream health care providers, they "address the root cause" of the problem and "treat the whole person." Ironically, they often do neither while the latter do both. Recall from Chapter 3 that a trope is a recurring, even overused, phrase, idea, or theme. Ernst has helped to uncover the common tropes of alternative medicine. Perhaps unsurprisingly, these same tropes are used in the alternative medicine community to sow distrust in mainstream mental health care and to market products and services related to mental health and illness. Drawing from the literature on this topic, I've compiled a nonexhaustive list that I urge you to read under the heading "Alternative Medicine Tropes and Corrections" on pages 202–205 in "Mind the Takeaways." Like the students in Trecek-King's class, you'll soon be unable to unsee these tropes.

The very existence of alternative medicine as a marketing campaign is predicated on creating a false dichotomy with mainstream health care—they are not two equal but different members of the same family. By definition, alternative medicine falls outside the purview of evidence-based medicine. As the comedian Tim Minchin famously asked: "Do you know what they call alternative medicine that's been proved to work? Medicine." That's because skepticism doesn't discriminate. The same level of incisive scientific scrutiny needs to be applied across health care disciplines. Unfortunately, alternative medicine inherently elevates pseudoscience in its commercial form as part of the wellness industry; it's a front for selling the fruits of fake science. To succeed, a polarizing narrative is required to perpetuate mistrust in health care that's never out of vogue.

But to paraphrase Winston Churchill's quip regarding democracy, evidence-based health care is the worst form of health care except for all those other forms that have been tried. While mistrust in science and health care can be well earned, the wellness industry uses alternative medicine to amplify and profit from that mistrust at the expense of our mental health.

Insidious Tactics

When I was a graduate student, I was invited by my research supervisor to coauthor a scientific review article about gambling disorders. My supervisor, David C. Hodgins, was (and still is) an internationally recognized leader in research investigating the nature and treatment of addiction. It wasn't the first time that he invited me to coauthor a scientific article, but this one was special. This article was to appear in *The Lancet*, which official rankings have considered to be the most influential medical journal in the world. I was ecstatic. At the time, I considered myself to be a lowly student unworthy of such an honor and opportunity. But I seized it, we published the article, and I ended up paying for my own hard copy of the journal issue to give to my cheerleading parents—who were surprised *The Lancet* wasn't paying us.

Many people don't realize that academic researchers aren't paid by the scientific journals that publish their work. They might also not realize that journals vary widely in quality, from top medical journals like *The Lancet* to pseudoscientific and even predatory journals that bypass the peer review process and charge author fees to publish. My spam email inbox is replete with polite invitations from predatory publishers requesting manuscript submissions, sometimes in domains outside of my expertise, and often containing spelling and grammar errors. Pseudoscientific journals are insidious: They may not always prey upon the wallets of unsuspecting professors, but they are governed by pseudoscientific red flags.

The journal *Explore* is one example. Recent issues contain studies on mediumship, after-death communication, essential oils, etc., all with results that confirm pseudoscientific hypotheses. I read one double-blind randomized controlled trial claiming to support the hypothesis that sending positive vibes to water can make its ice crystals look more beautiful.

There are countless pseudoscientific journals and studies. In the *Journal of Evidence-Based Complementary & Alternative Medicine*, you can read about a randomized controlled trial suggesting that prayer can reduce migraine headache pain without any mention of the placebo effect as a probable explanation for the results. In *The Journal of Alternative and Complementary Medicine*, it's said that practitioners can use Reiki to improve the growth of bacterial cultures, particularly if they score high on a measure of emotional well-being. And in the *Journal of Religion and Health*, you can find the argument that "it is time for medical professions to consider the possibility of demonic possession in the etiology of schizophrenia, especially in the cases with hallucinations and delusions."

Pseudoscientific journals legitimize bogus science by serving as a trusted conduit for misinformation used to buttress alternative medicine grift. Though they represent perhaps the most insidious yet impactful way that promoters of alternative medicine justify pseudoscientific approaches to mental health care, other propaganda tactics aid in the endeavor. I've included a list under the heading "Alternative Medicine Propaganda Tactics" on page 206 in "Mind the Takeaways."

* * *

The Amazing James Randi earned himself cult status in the skeptic community as a stage magician and author who made a career out of investigating and debunking pseudoscientific claims. He once said that "Magicians are the most honest people in the world; they tell you they're gonna fool you, and then they do it." The same can't be said of alternative medicine practitioners, who might not even be aware that they're fooling you, or themselves, or of the tropes and tactics they brandish.

Like Randi, Lilienfeld's leadership too left an indelible legacy. He wanted clinicians in the mental health professions to be more science informed in their practice and refused to let pseudoscience define psychology. He ventured into the philosophy of science to extract, translate, and teach how we might best identify pseudoscientific grift. Others have joined him in his efforts.

Yet, here we are today, living in a digital, cultural ecosystem that grows and sells charlatanry, a dynamic, worldwide mental health care space where someone like the Medical Medium can earn Hollywood celebrity accolades with bestselling books and detoxes that couldn't be more shamelessly informed by pseudoscience.

We've been given the tools to find and name the fraud. They exist in the scientific literature and can be effectively taught in the classroom. Our mental health can't afford for them to become lost relics. They're available—but they need to be accessed and applied.

So what gets in the way? Why can't we just drop lists from the sky that rain down like confetti that contain the pseudoscientific red flags or alternative medicine tropes and expect that people's mental health will be immune from exploitation? It turns out that protecting ourselves is not so easy.

Even with those lists in hand, we can still fall for fake scientific claims and misinformation. It's not just a matter of science and mental health literacy, or even pseudoscience literacy, though those skills are necessary. We also need to understand and become more cognizant of the psychological and social influences on our thinking and mental health decisions.

6

Falling for Fake Science News

At her sister's wedding in 2009, Kirby Brown couldn't contain her enthusiasm for a new self-help book she'd seen featured on *Oprah*. The bestseller was called *The Secret*, authored by Rhonda Byrne, based on a documentary film of the same name. Kirby raved to her sister about how one charismatic narrator in the film version had caught her eye. She felt connected to him. His name was James Arthur Ray. In addition to his frequent appearances on *Oprah*, he'd been touring on numerous other media venues, such as CNN's *Larry King Live* and the *Today Show*.

Kirby was an adventurer and the life and breath of the party. When her sister lived in Thailand, Kirby was the kind of person who went to visit her. Twice. Spiritually inclined, Kirby was also constantly yearning to learn, wanting to expand her decorative painting business in San Jose del Cabo, Mexico, and to grow on a personal level. When James advertised a free wellness event to give a taste of his teachings in Baja, Mexico, she didn't skip a beat.

More wellness events followed. Kirby even recruited her parents, who were both clinical social workers. She invited her mother to one in New Jersey, and at that event they enrolled her father for one in California. Her parents knew that the messages promoted at these events were not backed by science, but that mattered less than bonding with their daughter.

In October 2009, Kirby attended James's Spiritual Warrior wellness retreat in Sedona, Arizona. This was a 5-day intensive experience at a cost of $10,000 per person. Upon arrival, more than 50 participants were asked by James to shave their heads as a way to coalesce as a group. Later, they underwent deprivation exercises of various sorts, meditating in the desert without food, water, and sleep. They were told that if they were serious about their personal growth, then they needed to invest in themselves and expect pain and discomfort by partaking in a slew of physically and emotionally demanding activities.

The final day of the retreat culminated in what James called his *sweat lodge*. Participants crowded into a wood-frame dome draped with tarps and blankets, stooping under the low ceiling into a dark, windowless space around a pit filled with heated stones. A heavy tarp door was the only way in and out and the only source of light and oxygen. The sweat lodge was James's final test, representing a symbolic death in a feat of personal transformation. According to several participants, he said, "You are not going to die. You might think you are, but you are not going to die."

A few hours after participants entered the dome, the harm couldn't be ignored any longer. People were vomiting and crying. Others were dazed and delirious. One person had even fallen into the heated stones, burning his arm. Emergency responders were eventually called and they performed CPR on at least three unconscious participants.

At 38 years old, Kirby was among those found unconscious. She died from heatstroke. Another participant, James Shore, also died from heatstroke, and a third, Liz Neuman, slipped into a coma and died 9 days later from organ failure. Eighteen other participants were hospitalized for various health problems, including dehydration, burns, kidney failure, breathing difficulties, and heat exhaustion. In the introduction of James's 2020 book, *The Business of Redemption: The Price of Leadership in Both Life and Business*, he recounts those moments:

> Within the hour, as police and emergency vehicles swarmed the area, I would hear a detective say, "Mr. Ray, I hope you know we're investigating this as a homicide." Everything went silent. I glanced over at the sweat lodge; they had already roped off the area with yellow crime scene tape. A homicide? "Look, you might go to jail tonight," a criminal lawyer told me later that evening. "If you do, we'll get you out as soon as we can." Jail? Are you kidding me? My head was spinning fast, and I thought I just might throw up.

James was found guilty of three counts of negligent homicide in November 2011 and sentenced to 2 years in prison. He served 20 months.

Since leaving prison he has re-entered the wellness space, casting himself as a life coach. He has been interviewed by Larry King's successor, Piers Morgan, who on CNN's *Piers Morgan Live* suggested, "You could be in an even better position now to help people who had been through a nightmarish experience." James also starred in a documentary called *Enlighten Us* that appeared on Netflix. On his website, he still markets himself as a multi-bestselling author and contributor to *The Secret*, offering personal growth consulting services and selling courses for thousands of dollars a pop. The description of one course, called "Quantum Leap," indicates that it can change your life in several ways: "You'll vanquish fears and anxiety that keep you paralyzed; All the anger that blurs your visions and keeps you from thinking straight will literally melt away; You'll put the past in the past and drop grief and guilt like a hot potato." There's even a section of his website devoted to the "Sedona Sweat Lodge." It contains the introduction of his new book, detailing how he has incorporated the incident at Spiritual Warrior into his own redemption story of personal growth to teach about leadership skills. Of course, there's also a link to where the book can be purchased.

* * *

You might be wondering: How do people get sucked into these kinds of charades—smart, intelligent people, like you and me, and Kirby? It's one thing to read and believe misinformation—it's an order of magnitude worse when that misinformation steers decisions about our mental health.

By now, James's wellness grift may feel palpable to you. While it's becoming increasingly recognized that sweat lodge ceremonies could be an important aspect of culturally competent Indigenous healing, James had no idea what he was doing. He didn't have the years of training in ceremonial knowledge that are required by traditional spiritual leaders who are recognized by their community to safely facilitate such a high-risk event. Unqualified to provide interventions related to mental health, he also drew from pseudoscientific treatments and ideas to inform his approach, such as neurolinguistic programming (to be exposed in the next chapter) and *The Secret*'s "law of attraction." Recall from Chapter 2 that the law of attraction is scientifically implausible and unhelpful to people who experience obsessive-compulsive disorder and anxiety disorders. It posits that if we focus our thoughts on something we wish to obtain, then it will come to us.

In 2020, the same year that James published his redemption story, Kirby's mother and sister copublished their own book entitled *This Sweet Life: How We Lived After Kirby Died*. They relay how they discovered her death, how they grieved, what it was like to live through James's trial, and how they survived the aftermath. I reached out to Kirby's sister, Jean Brown, to learn more about Kirby, to renew her voice, and to illustrate some concepts related to our susceptibility to misinformation. What follows is a truncated version of our interview:

STEA: What made James Ray compelling and dangerous?

BROWN: Kirby got into his ecosystem quicky. It was the fact that he seemed so legitimate. The media legitimized him. He was involved in *The Secret*, *Oprah*, and the *Today Show*. He was charming and people listened to him. At the Spiritual Warrior event, people did what he said, and the activities broke them down. They couldn't say "no." They were told to ignore their signs of discomfort and to expect it, including heatstroke. We can see the warning signs now in retrospect. But we didn't know them at the time. My sister didn't know. What's dangerous about him now is the spinning of the tragedy for his own gain, spinning reality to suit his own narrative. We can see the harm caused by people like him in the wellness industry. People may say, "Well, I enjoy such wellness activities and it's good for me," but that doesn't negate from the fact that it's potentially very harmful.

STEA: What's your understanding of how amazing, intelligent people like Kirby fall for his grift?

BROWN: People who wouldn't think they are susceptible can get pulled in. We are all vulnerable. That said, some types of people are more at risk, particularly those who are in a period of change or making a big transition in their life, such as people in recovery from addiction and mental health problems, or college age people—basically, people who are motivated and open to new experiences and ideas. Seeking personal growth requires a kind of vulnerability and openness and ability to change beliefs and values. But vulnerability is not weakness. Kirby was a force of nature. No one that knew her would describe her as weak. She was determined. She was motivated to make a change in her life. That motivation makes people push through, especially when a guru or leader is telling you to keep going.

STEA: How did James target his victims?

BROWN: They offer free wellness events. Once you're at an event, then comes the heavy sales pitch to sign up for the next course. At these events, you might hear about five wellness ideas. Two of them may seem okay, like good ideas that are repackaged from stuff that works, and the other three ideas are really out there and far fetched. They use other tactics too. Some of them are cult-y. Like at the Spiritual Warrior event, they first had to shave their heads. It disconnects people from their identity and creates bonding. The deprivation exercises make people weaker so they're more at the whim of the leader. "Love bombing" occurs too, which means showering you with compliments and making you feel amazing. When all of this happens, people feel like they have a transformative experience that convinces them it's working and they need to do more and more. They're on a high from the event.

STEA: How would you describe Kirby's legacy?

BROWN: Her story is a cautionary tale. Having strong people meet their end at an event like that was so shocking to many people. She was strong, like physically strong—she lived in Mexico and was used to the heat. To have someone so strong meet her end in a physical way was shocking. She was only 38. I just really want people to know who she was. She had a zest for life. She was willing to live unconventionally. She was spiritual. She was able to hold on to all of these things and was very fun, and caring, and a rock for many of her friends—someone people would turn to in times of crisis.

Kirby's cautionary tale is unfortunately not unique to her. These kinds of stories of harm, even in their fatal extremity, are unnecessary and worldwide. An eerily similar case in China involved the death of 32-year-old Sara Wei; a 2021 news headline read: "Life Coaching Takes a Deadly Turn After Young Executive Dies Following $14,000-Course That Amplifies Negative Emotions and Targets Participants' Mental Demons by Evoking Past Traumas." Another case in England involved the death of 32-year-old Kate Hyatt, with a 2023 headline reading: "Artist, 32, Took Her Own Life After Drinking Hallucinogenic 'Tea' in Trendy Shamanic Healing Ritual at £620-a-Head Retreat, Inquest Hears."

I think Kirby's mother, Ginny Brown, put it best when she was quoted as saying: "It's just terrible that our daughter had to die before we could see how dangerous someone like James Ray really could be. But this is bigger than James Ray. This is bigger than our daughter."

The answer to the question, of how people fall for grift, is not at all straightforward. It's multidimensional. When we look to the rich, emerging scientific literature on this topic, we see that it's incredibly convoluted and can be best understood by considering the interaction of many different reasons. Let's walk through some of those reasons now.

Nobel Disease

In the 1660s, Sir Isaac Newton invented an entire branch of math called calculus. He was among the most brilliant scientists who ever lived, but he was also preoccupied with strange spiritual ideas, such as extracting prophecies from secret biblical codes. Sir Arthur Conan Doyle lived over two centuries later as a physician and author of the fictional detective Sherlock Holmes, who is an icon of critical thinking in popular culture. Doyle also fell for the Cottingley Fairies hoax in the early 20th century, in which two cousins faked five photographs depicting them in a garden surrounded by small fairies. Alfred Russel Wallace codiscovered the theory of evolution by natural selection in the mid- to late 1800s, along with Charles Darwin. Wallace also believed in ghosts, loved phrenology—the pseudoscientific attempt to understand mental life by linking personality traits with skull shape—and was an anti-vaccine extremist. More recently, Ben Carson, a retired neurosurgeon and politician with more than 60 honorary doctorate degrees, has advocated for untested herbal supplements as a cancer treatment and maintained that the Egyptian pyramids were constructed to store grain, contrary to historical expertise.

In 2001, the British geneticist Paul Nurse won the Nobel Prize in Physiology or Medicine along with Leland Hartwell and Tim Hunt for their discoveries of protein molecules that control the division of cells in the cell cycle. And in 2013, he issued a plea to future Nobel Prize recipients that could've equally served as a caution to the otherwise impressive scientists above. Nurse warned against "believing you are expert in almost everything . . . or you will be in danger of succumbing to Nobelitis."

We learned in Chapter 2 that no matter how scientifically literate you are, you can still be duped by peddlers of pseudoscience. Research shows that science literacy doesn't always directly translate to better health behaviors because there are so many other variables at play. The stories of Newton, Doyle, Wallace, and Carson attest to the idea that the most scientifically literate and intelligent people can in some instances think and behave in the most unscientific and unintelligent ways. There's a name for this affliction: It's called Nobel disease, or as Nurse dubbed it, Nobelitis. The name comes from the observation that a surprising number of scientific Nobel Prize recipients fall prey to some obvious examples of misinformation.

It's unknown whether Nobel Prize winners are more prone to this tendency than other people, including scientists. Some researchers believe that

Nobel disease can partly be explained by a kind of "guru complex," whereby once scientists achieve "guru" status by virtue of their accomplishments, fame, and adoring acolytes, their self-perceptions may become distorted, leading them to overlook their limitations and publicly venture outside their domains of expertise to foolishly opine on matters they don't understand.

The point is that while science literacy, critical thinking, and intelligence are definitely important with respect to not succumbing to misinformation, they're only part of the puzzle. Other variables matter too, such as intellectual humility, which can be thought of as a propensity to be aware of our own personal biases and limitations. Recall the study described in Chapter 2 when researchers found that no matter the topic, people who disagreed most with the scientific consensus knew less about it but thought they knew more. Remaining intellectually humble is one key antidote to rejecting the consensus of an overwhelming body of scientific studies that agree with and support each other.

While learning to trust expertise is easier for some people than others, and for good reason, the reality is that trusting the expertise that informs evidence-based mental health care is another important way to lessen the risk of getting duped. According to a 2021 study, people who were susceptible to online misinformation about one health topic were likely to be susceptible to many types of health misinformation, and those who were most susceptible had less education and health literacy, less faith in the health care system, and more positive attitudes toward alternative medicine. Yes, we need to prudently walk the line between trusting expertise and holding healthy scientific skepticism. At the same time, we cannot afford to let mistrust completely rule our mental health decisions.

We Think in Shortcuts, Not Algorithms

On social media, I've received messages from people telling me that they feel embarrassed for falling for mental health scams. They beat themselves up, wondering how they were tricked. They'll exclaim something like, "I'm smarter than that!" They also feel validated when they learn that people are scammed for reasons other than their intelligence. It's a relief to learn that research shows we are all prone to errors in thinking that leave us vulnerable to misinformation.

A human brain that's home to an average of 86 billion neurons makes it impossible to track and analyze every single piece of past and present information in our environment. It's just too taxing. Instead, our brains evolved to color information with past experiences and have become wired for shortcuts to make it easier to efficiently navigate our world. In the history of our species, using these mental shortcuts provided our ancestors with an evolutionary advantage. Most of the time, they work. Other times, they function as biases and get us into trouble by causing us to overlook critical information.

The scientific method is a toolbox of techniques designed to counter our ingrained thinking tendencies and minimize human error. But we don't have the scientific method at our disposal in everyday life, such as when we're deciding what mental health information to believe or what decisions to make about our care. Instead, we need to rely on our science and mental health literacy skills and approach matters of evidence with critical thinking and humility. To remain intellectually humble, it helps to know and understand what common thinking errors look like so that we can learn to tune into and upset these biases that filter the way we see the world. I've included a nonexhaustive list of common thinking errors (sometimes referred to as cognitive biases) that are relevant to protection from mental health pseudoscience and misinformation in "Mind the Takeaways" under the heading "Common Thinking Errors (Cognitive Biases)" on pages 207–208.

It turns out that no matter how smart we are, the default setting of our brains is to think heuristically. Research shows that intelligence tends to be largely uncorrelated with most cognitive biases, such as base rate neglect (i.e., *neglecting or ignoring statistical information in favor of information pertaining to only a specific case*), belief bias (i.e., *judging the strength of an argument based on how plausible the conclusion sounds rather than the strength of its premises*), and confirmation bias (i.e., *seeking out evidence consistent with our beliefs and denying or distorting evidence that doesn't fit with our beliefs*). This means that even highly intelligent people can fail to think critically about information, especially when they aren't motivated to do so and believe they're right. In fact, some research even shows that intelligent people may have a somewhat larger bias blind spot (i.e., *believing that it's other people who are prone to cognitive biases while remaining blind to our own*) than others, meaning that the smartest people may be less aware of their own biases.

At the end of the day, there is no cure for thinking errors. We're stuck with them. But knowing them can assist with cultivating our intellectual humility and help us spot how grifters exploit the way we think. In the previous chapter, we learned about various alternative medicine tropes used to target our mental health. Some of these tropes assume the form of logical fallacies—which are also thinking errors—to capitalize on our tendency toward lazy thinking. Put differently, logical fallacies are persuasively packaged and used by proponents of alternative medicine to sing to our biases—not our intellects. Understanding these fallacies gives our intellects a chance to fight back.

I've listed some of the ways grifters appeal to our biases under the heading "Logical Fallacies Used to Promote Alternative Medicine" on pages 208–210 in "Mind the Takeaways."

Brightly Blinded by Belief

Imagine hopping on a plane and traveling to the beautiful country of Croatia. Before you start sightseeing, however, your destination is to join up to 10,000 people per day to cure your mental health concerns by visiting a "Super Healer" named Braco, born Josip Grbavac. Your visit is unlike your experience with other health care providers. There is no assessment and no treatment plan. There is no sales pitch for a "wellness event," thankfully. This time, you won't even have a conversation. Instead, you will corral with other like-minded people into an auditorium to bear witness to Braco's silent gaze for a 10- to 15-minute session. That's all. Staring at you and his audience from a podium has earned Braco the trusting eyes of people who pay to be in his presence. It might sound preposterous and extreme, but people have been falling for his grift since 1995. While he has a website disclaimer noting that he doesn't provide diagnoses or treatment, his advertising claims that he's "earned a reputation as one of Europe's most influential healers."

I had to gaze into Braco's eyes for myself. While the prospect of flying to Croatia was certainly appealing, it was easier and cheaper to livestream one of his 13 daily gazing sessions, freely available online from his website. The session began by playing soul-soothing New Age music followed by a hyped introduction by a member of Braco's public relations team. "They feel something though Braco's gaze," said his team. "When he stands in front of groups of people, they feel a sense of hope. They feel peace. They feel like life makes sense again."

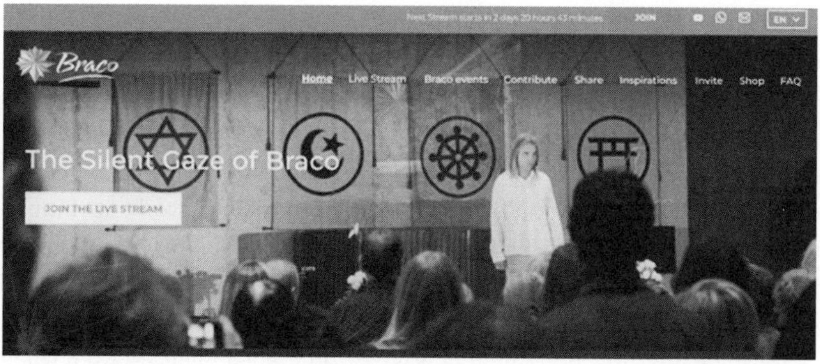

After his team primes viewers for what to expect, a short video is played depicting tearful observers yearning for hope and comfort. Braco then takes the stage, backlit by a human-sized, golden 13-ray sun symbol. The sun is his logo, representing "connection to that which Braco shares through his gaze." It can also be purchased as jewelry at his events, such as a 14-karat gold pendant for $5,000 and a diamond-encrusted 24-karat gold version for $9,000. As we gazed into each other's eyes during the livestream through my laptop, I tried really hard to just let go and give in to the process. I immediately noticed his warm, slightly watery eyes and barely perceptible, gentle smile as he stood rocking back and forth ever so subtly. It was a captivating experience. He made me feel like I wanted to get to know him, which is perhaps unsurprising in light of research showing that direct gazing among strangers can induce thoughts and feelings related to social bonding.

But the science stops there. There's no evidence that Braco's kind of gazing has any health benefits at all, despite testimonials on his website claiming that he's been able to heal everything from posttraumatic stress disorder to cancer. How might Braco's followers justify their belief in his abilities?

This is a loaded question, to be sure, but one variable involved in convincing people to buy into such weird ideas is called *motivated reasoning*. It essentially refers to an unconscious tendency to make information fit in a way that justifies a desired belief. Metaphorically, it's mental gymnastics, a kind of ideological blindness. When we engage in motivated reasoning, we begin with a conclusion that we want to believe, and then, unintentionally and unknowingly, we reason backward to convince ourselves that it's correct.

When it comes to Braco, it's possible that some of his devotees believe in his abilities regardless of whether evidence is shown that his method is a scientifically implausible way to treat any health condition, including mental illness. Some might reason, as they have in testimonials on his website, that one just needs to "open your heart to it," or that "what Braco does is beyond our imagination and beyond perception because it is God's work, not human work," or that "the number of people who come to see Braco, looking for help, certainly indicates how valuable he is."

Decades of research on the topic of motivated reasoning describe how facts can be interpreted in different ways, by different audiences. Even when we aren't blind to the facts because they're given to us, we may still process and interpret those facts in ways consistent with our preexisting values and beliefs. Think of Democrats and Republicans who "hate-read" the exact same news story about each other.

For example, some experiments have shown that even when people do possess accurate knowledge about the scientific consensus on a given topic, such as the reality of human evolution, they may nonetheless refuse to *know* it—meaning they will not integrate that knowledge into their attitudes, beliefs, or policy preferences. In this way, rejection of scientific consensus sometimes doesn't reflect a lack of information but instead motivated reasoning against that information. There's also evidence suggesting that motivated reasoning is most likely to occur when emotions are high, such as feeling angry, and among people with high intelligence and who have the most sophistication and knowledge of the topic. Thinking back to Nobel disease, maybe it's unsurprising that extremely smart people may be especially skilled at convincing themselves that their foolish beliefs are true. Ultimately, motivated reasoning, like cognitive biases, can contribute to a person becoming misinformed even when processing valid information.

Openness to Pseudo-Profound Bullshit and Conspiracies

If you traverse the pseudoscientific lands of the wellness industry on a regular basis, then you might detect a certain peculiarity in the way language is presented and understood. Scattered among alternative medicine social media groups, in-person events, online forums, and practitioner websites are bullshit statements that people believe, consisting of buzzwords and phrases with no discernible meaning. They sound something like this: "Wholeness quiets infinite phenomena," or "We are in the midst of a high-frequency blossoming of interconnectedness that will give us access to the quantum soup itself."

Those particular statements were generated by cognitive psychologist Gordon Pennycook and his fellow researchers as part of their interest in studying this phenomenon more broadly. They famously called it *pseudo-profound bullshit*, which describes the tendency to perceive superficially deep but vacuous assertions as meaningful. And for their efforts, they won the most amusingly insightful and coveted distinction in the world of science: the Ig Nobel Prize.

Held annually at Harvard University, the ceremony for the Ig Nobel Prize celebrates scientific achievements that "first make people laugh and then make them think." While it's a satirical award, it's handed out by actual Nobel laureates. Other winners along with Pennycook and his team included German scientists who revealed that people could relieve itches on their left forearm by looking into the mirror and scratching their right forearm, and the late Egyptian urologist Ahmed Shafik, who studied the effects of wearing polyester, cotton, or wool trousers on the sex lives of rats.

While unusual, Pennycook's research has been pivotal in understanding how people detect and believe pseudoscientific claims. "Our work shows how readily people accept claims that sound good (or feel good), but that are actually empty or meaningless," he told me. His team showed, for example, that people have a tough time telling the difference between made-up bullshit statements (e.g., "hidden meaning transforms unparalleled abstract beauty") and the actual X (formerly Twitter) feed of Deepak Chopra (e.g., "attention and intention are the mechanics of manifestation"), just one wellness guru among many who speaks with vagueness and ambiguity to mask and market baloney ideas. Chopra has written over 20 *New York Times* bestsellers and has over 3 million followers on X (formerly Twitter). As we're well aware, bullshit is popular.

Across multiple studies, Pennycook's team also demonstrated that people who were more receptive to pseudo-profound bullshit tended to be lower in intelligence, more prone to conspiracy thinking, more likely to hold religious and paranormal beliefs, and more likely to believe that alternative medicine works. Crucially, they also found that people who more easily fell for pseudo-profound bullshit relied more on an intuitive style of thinking that feels impulsive, emotional, and automatic rather than a style of thinking that is more deliberate and effortful, called analytical thinking. In other words, critical thinking matters. Pennycook told me that "those who are more willing to actually question their intuitions by engaging in reflection are less vulnerable to misinformation and other forms of bullshitting." This is consistent with decades of scientific research stemming partly from the pioneering work of Nobel Prize recipient Daniel Kahneman, who once said, "Delay your intuition. Slow down. Sleep on it. Break the problem into smaller parts." (Incidentally, I once asked Kahneman to be involved in a book that I coedited, and he graciously declined, citing his lack of expertise on the subject. When I contrast his humility with the daily death of expertise on social media, I die a little inside. He certainly doesn't suffer from Nobel disease.)

Our psychology can also influence our health beliefs in other ways. Recall that we're evolutionarily wired for mental shortcuts because it helps us to efficiently navigate our world without burdening the brain with the need to attend to and analyze every single source of incoming information. Our minds have adapted in this way to seek out and detect patterns that help us avoid danger and make sense of our noisy, chaotic environments. Evolution has favored this tendency, but it can also lead us awry. This means that we're all prone to seeing order in disorder and meaning in meaninglessness—even when there really isn't any.

For example, we see objects and faces in clouds, and some of us look to astrological horoscopes to give us a sense of control and predictability in an unpredictable world. Rigorous studies have revealed that when we lack a sense of control, our tendency to detect patterns is heightened, even when the patterns we find are random and don't exist. This psychological phenomenon is known as *illusory pattern perception* and helps to explain why lacking control makes people much more likely to believe in paranormal activity, superstitious thinking, and conspiracies. When our minds re-establish control by finding patterns and meaning, life can feel more predictable, less anxiety provoking, and less aversive.

You might be unsurprised to learn about evidence suggesting that those of us who have a greater tendency to detect illusory patterns are also more likely to be receptive to pseudo-profound bullshit. So it's no wonder that many of us are drawn to pseudoscientific claims, such as *The Secret*'s law of attraction or Braco's purported healing abilities. We all wish to have greater control over our lives, and some of us just have a greater propensity to make sense from nonsense than others.

Sometimes that propensity manifests in extreme ways and impacts our health behaviors. People who believe in conspiracy theories are convinced that particular events can be explained by the secret plots of two or more powerful actors. And believing conspiracies is more common than we might think.

Even back in 2014, before we all experienced a sense of lack of control associated with the Covid-19 pandemic, the prestigious medical journal *JAMA* (*Journal of the American Medical Association*) reported that about half of Americans agreed with at least one medical conspiracy, such as "doctors and the government still want to vaccinate children even though they know these vaccines cause autism and other psychological disorders." In that study, people who tended to believe such conspiracies were also more likely to report avoidance of evidence-based health care and greater use of alternative medicine. This makes sense when we consider evidence that mistrust of institutions and health care providers is one underlying common denominator of both believing in conspiracies and using alternative medicine.

Some scientists have suggested that there may be such a thing as a general tendency toward conspiracy thinking, called *conspiracy mentality*. This is because people who believe in conspiracies typically believe in more than just one, even when they're unrelated. The physiologist Mark Hoofnagle noticed this too and coarsely used the term *crank magnetism* to describe the phenomenon where—like a magnet—belief in one type of pseudoscience or conspiracy tends to attract multiple types. This tracks with the scientific literature, further reinforcing the story we've been unpacking all along: No matter the details of particular pseudoscientific claims or conspiracies, some of us are pulled in due to our underlying traits, such as differences in our tendencies toward believing pseudo-profound bullshit and conspiracy thinking.

Another key component of our psychological makeup matters here too. Personality psychologists have found that a trait called *openness to experience* is strongly linked to people using alternative medicine and believing its claims. It refers to people who would describe themselves as curious, open-minded, and attracted to new experiences. Researchers have found that people who score higher in openness to experience tend to rely more on intuitive thinking (as opposed to analytical thinking) and to be more vaccine hesitant. This jibes with evidence that those who rely on intuitive thinking are more likely to be receptive to pseudo-profound bullshit and buy into alternative medicine claims. Like all personality traits, openness to experience is a double-edged sword. Extremely high levels can produce awe-inspiring feats of creativity but also place some at risk for trusting outrageous ideas.

Targeting Biases on Steroids

For better or worse, I've spent way too much time on social media. You probably have too. It's built into the fabric of our culture. I can't tell you how many times my therapy patients have wanted to address social media use as part of their treatment goals. Some merely want to limit their use, while others are concerned about the way in which interactions negatively impact their mental health, particularly when discussing emotionally charged topics, such as politics. Still others come to me with questions about mental health information that they read or were told online. "Does cannabis actually help with anxiety? Are psychedelics really a cure for addiction? Do antidepressants work at all? Is naturopathy completely safe? If I change my diet, will my depression just go away?"

It's no conspiracy to say that social media is a breeding ground for misinformation. Ongoing bodies of research are piecing together the moving parts of exactly what makes it fertile. We know, for instance, that as social creatures, we often fragment into groups both offline and online. An unhelpful by-product of this fragmentation is that it can create online bubbles or echo chambers that filter out some kinds of information and socially reward the sharing of other kinds. Psychiatrist Joe Pierre has referred to these echo chambers as confirmation bias on steroids. They can teach us to reject information that we encounter from groups with whom we disagree and to fight tooth and nail to support our own convictions.

Echo chambers toy with our biases in other ways too. Inside them, we may not even see information that contradicts our beliefs. The homogeneity and repetitiveness of the information that we do see will feel more familiar and believable over time. Kahneman famously wrote that "a reliable way to make people believe in falsehoods is frequent repetition, because familiarity is not easily distinguished from truth." By exposing ourselves only to limited information shared by people with whom we agree, we allow echo chambers to play off and magnify our vulnerabilities to thinking errors beyond confirmation bias, including the availability heuristic (i.e., *relying on information that quickly comes to mind*), in-group bias (i.e., *unfairly favoring our own group*), and groupthink (i.e., *preoccupation with what the group thinks rather than critically evaluating the information at hand*).

The very structure of social media networks themselves poses another problem to receiving unbiased information. Research has shown that the algorithms of X (formerly Twitter) and Facebook work against us in ways that can lead some false information to be perceived as more common than it is in reality. This issue is worsened by the fact that bad actors (both human and machine-bots) do exist and can exploit the visibility of false information. At an even higher level of analysis, political and popular media conglomerates can be influenced to share what information is disseminated to the public, as their survival depends on competition for funding and public attention. I don't know how you feel, but this is disconcerting to me, especially given evidence that fake science news on X (formerly Twitter) spreads further, faster, and deeper than the truth.

I once interviewed Peter Hotez, a scientist who was nominated for the 2022 Nobel Peace Prize for his work in vaccine development and combating anti-vaccine propaganda. He told me, "It's important to recognize that many individuals who espouse anti-vaccine views are themselves victims who have been targeted with misinformation." The same could be said about mental health misinformation.

Scientists are just beginning to understand how other group and societal factors might inadvertently contribute to misinformation spread. For instance, decreasing public and policy support for science has incentivized scientific organizations, including psychological and psychiatric organizations, to use popular and social media to promote particular findings or kinds of research. Celebrity scientists speaking to mental health topics and journalists untrained in science journalism may be increasingly relied on as resources for newsworthy accounts of breakthrough science. This concerns me, and it should concern you too. It means that hyped-up, cherry-picked, inaccurate portrayals of research in press releases, news headlines, and other modes of communication can be amplified, making it easier for misinformation to be platformed to the public.

I spoke out against one such example by writing in the popular press in 2019 along with my colleague Tyler Marshall. We had both read a study demonstrating that a short-term course of cannabidiol (CBD)—one of many phytocannabinoid compounds found in the cannabis plant—reduced cue-induced cravings and anxiety in people who were abstinent from heroin but recovering from heroin addiction. Contrasting the specificity of those results with the hyperbolic headlines in popular media, such as *Rolling Stone* ("New Study Finds CBD Could Curb Heroin Addiction") and CNN ("Study Finds CBD Effective in Treating Heroin Addiction"), displayed a striking case of misinformation that we couldn't ignore, given the seriousness of the opioid crisis in North America.

Fortunately, it's not all doom and gloom. At a personal level, we can work against the social and popular media structures that are working against us. Publishing in *Nature*, Pennycook and his team showed that people on X (formerly Twitter) who were more likely to override intuitive thinking with analytical thinking were less gullible, less likely to exist in echo chambers, and less likely to spread fake science news. If we go beyond the headlines, prioritize awareness of our biases, and pause to think about the accuracy of content we encounter, then we're much better positioned to avoid getting sucked in by falsehoods.

###

When I reached out to Jean Brown to glean her insights about Kirby's story, I was deeply moved and inspired by her spirit, and her family's. We all fall for fake science news at times to varying degrees, and it's easier in hindsight to see what went wrong. The Brown family decided to turn their tragedy into something positive. They founded an organization called SEEK Safely (http://www.seeksafely.org) that is dedicated to educating the public about the potential harms of the wellness industry with a view toward empowering consumers and promoting safety and practitioner accountability through legislative action. Jean is the content producer.

She told me the organization wants to underscore that "There's nothing wrong with people seeking personal growth and deeper meaning, looking for ways to improve their mental health, and being open to new ideas and experiences. That's very valid. But we also want to help people understand that with that vulnerability comes the risk of being taken advantage of." On their website, they also have an initiative called the SEEK Safely Promise. It encourages wellness practitioners to sign a promise to publicly commit to safe practices, and in return, they would receive a printable certificate and badge to proudly use in their own marketing materials. Despite being asked by the family, James Ray has refused to sign it.

Fake science news will continue to be all around us. Understanding the reasons we fall for it can feel like getting lost in a labyrinth. It's normal to feel overwhelmed by its complexity. It can be helpful to think about what's in our control. The majority of us can't do anything about the algorithms of X (formerly Twitter) or the way tainted mental health information is presented in popular media. Rather, we can pay attention to our own unique risk factors and do our best to mitigate them by cultivating intellectual humility, remembering our favorite thinking errors, pinpointing logical fallacies in alternative medicine advertising, gaining self-understanding about our personalities, and critically thinking about information, especially if it looks like pseudo-profound bullshit. This awareness is our friend when trying to figure out the legitimacy of particular mental health–related assessments, diagnoses, and treatments, which we turn to now.

7

Exposing Bunk

Inaccurate Assessments and Bogus Treatments

Picture this: Your loved one has been missing work lately. Sleeping through the night has always been difficult, but it's become much worse for them during the past few weeks. They frequently wake up in a sweating panic and tell you afterward about these vivid, incessant nightmares that keep them too frightened to go back to sleep. At the grocery store, they suddenly jump and scream in the checkout line because a stranger inadvertently touched their back when placing their food on the conveyer belt. It's like they have an exaggerated startle reflex. Several such incidents have happened recently, causing them to profusely apologize and feel embarrassed—and so their world has been shrinking more and more as they refuse to go out in public.

For the first time in a long time, thoughts of suicide have crept back into their daydreams. Fearing further mental deterioration, they reach out to you for help. You discover that a new employee at their work setting reminds them of their abusive childhood they've tried to forget. Your loved one has been skipping work not only due to exhaustion but also to avoid any thoughts and memories related to this new employee. You decide to take them to the hospital because you're especially worried about their suicidal thoughts. Following a psychiatric evaluation, you learn that their symptoms are consistent with a diagnosis of posttraumatic stress disorder (PTSD). Your loved one is sent home after 3 days because their suicidal thoughts have dampened. In conjunction with medication, you've both been advised that the next step is to seek outpatient psychotherapy for PTSD.

Unsure about where to look, a close friend suggests exploring something called past life regression therapy. They just finished reading a book about it involving the case of a patient named Catherine who expressed similar symptoms to your loved one. "[Catherine] was suffering from fears, phobias, paralyzing panic attacks, depression, and recurrent nightmares," described the book, *Through Time Into Healing: Discovering the Power of Regression Therapy to Erase Trauma and Transform Mind, Body, and Relationships.*

So you do more digging. You learn that the book was written by an Ivy League–trained psychiatrist named Brian L. Weiss, who published at least 10 books on past life regression therapy and related subjects. One of those books, *Many Lives, Many Masters*, sold over a million copies. Lending further legitimacy to this avenue, you find that celebrity physician Dr. Oz has praised Weiss's methods and that Oprah's Emmy Award–winning series, *Super Soul Sunday*, featured an episode depicting how Weiss effectively treated Catherine's symptoms. It details how Weiss hypnotized Catherine to remember "repressed and forgotten traumas" not only from her childhood but also from three past lives: one as a "near-Eastern" woman who died in a flood about 4,000 years ago, a second as a Greek woman who lived a few hundred years after the near-Eastern lifetime, and a third as a "Spanish prostitute" in the 18th century.

You think to yourself, "Seriously? Past lives?" So you buy Weiss's book to understand more and then read: "Week by week, [Catherine's] formerly intractable symptoms disappeared as under hypnosis she remembered more past lives. Within a few months she was totally cured, without the use of any medicines."

Wanting your loved one to experience the same relief as Catherine, you Google "past life regression therapy" in your local area and find numerous providers who offer the service, most of whom are not licensed mental health professionals but boast certificates obtained from attending multiday hypnotherapy workshops. You hop on social media and become one of more than 255 million viewers to click the TikTok hashtag #pastliferegression. It leads you to watch videos of people recounting both positive and negative experiences in response to a 36-minute YouTube clip of Weiss directing a recorded past life regression session. An article in the *New York Times* then comes across your search giving space to at least one practitioner who discloses that she alone has conducted several thousand past life regressions.

"Why not?" you wonder. Desperation is setting in and your loved one has always had a spiritual bent to them anyway. You book an initial appointment for $250.

* * *

If this scenario were real, then the fate of your loved one would unlikely be their death. But they wouldn't receive safe, ethical, competent care either. Past life regression therapy is based on the reincarnation hypothesis and is used to treat mental health concerns by addressing events that an individual went through before they were born in this life. There's no plausible scientific theory or body of evidence supporting its use. Like with any pseudoscientific treatment—as we'll discuss in Chapter 8—people can report benefits due to a number of reasons other than the therapy itself, including the placebo effect and factors that are common across all talk therapies, such as the experience of being heard and validated by a clinician. This doesn't negate from the clinical reality: Not only could seeking past life regression therapy delay effective treatment, but also it has the potential to be directly harmful.

We know, for instance, that a strong body of scientific research supports the idea that memory is malleable. Many people assume that memory works like a tape on which events are recorded objectively from start to finish. The reality is much wonkier because the way we remember events has numerous influences, such as our past experiences, mood, and verbal suggestion. Research has shown that we can remember events that never actually happened and that such false memories can even be implanted unintentionally.

For example, in the case of hypnosis and past life regression therapy, a clinician may ask, "Were you ever a seamstress in the Middle Ages?" Such leading questions, combined with expectations to satisfy a clinician, can result in a patient elaborating on the details. The mind fills in the blanks. This can feel like a real memory. It also opens the possibility that traumatic false memories from a previous life could be implanted too, especially among the estimated one-third of American adults who believe in reincarnation and the likely higher number of people in countries with religions (e.g., Hinduism) that include reincarnation as a facet of their belief systems.

I find it disconcerting that such an unmistakably pseudoscientific treatment like past life regression therapy is so ubiquitous and can easily be marketed toward people who experience mental disorders. To this day, Weiss leads mass past life regression sessions and offers 5-day training workshops for "therapists and non-therapists alike." He's told the *New York Times* that at one of these workshops, he drew more than 200 people into a "meditative state" and then encouraged them to walk through imaginary doors labeled with years such as 1850, 1700, 1500, and so on, to find past life memories. "Any good therapist can use these techniques and you can learn them in a week," he said.

More disconcerting is that past life regression therapy is not alone. There are an estimated 600 brands of psychotherapy circulating in the world of mental health, and that number is growing at a nauseating rate. The vast majority of these psychotherapies have never been subjected to randomized controlled trials and remain untested, with many accompanied by more fanfare than theoretical rationale. The hype overshadows the lack of evidence. While some of the therapies may indeed be effective, some may cause direct harm. We just don't know.

Later in this chapter, I want to survey with you some of the most popular pseudoscientific treatments that claim to address mental health concerns, as well as ones that reside in the gray zone. I can't address them all, but my grander hope is that you will apply the same critical lens I use to scrutinize these treatments to ones not covered. But before we can dive deeper into treatment, we need to talk about assessment.

Horoscopes for Nerds

After a long day of work, my wife and I like to indulge in a shameful habit: We watch reality TV. Occasionally, fashionable mental health scams appear on the screen, and I need to bite my tongue so that I don't annoy her with a tirade. Watching *The Kardashians* makes my tongue bleed.

I remember one episode when Khloe Kardashian and Kendall Jenner met psychiatrist Daniel G. Amen and his futuristic-looking blue brain scanner. "Kendall's got a beautiful brain on the outside," Amen said, as he pointed toward a computer screen with brightly colored images. "But if we look at her emotional brain, which is right here, it's way too busy, which is why she can struggle with anxiety." To Khloe, Amen revealed other details. He said, "You can be anxious. And you worry. And you have trauma. Do you see this diamond? So this will often go with emotional trauma." By the end of the episode, my brain hurt—figuratively of course.

Amen was assessing the mental health of the sisters using a brain imaging diagnostic tool called single-proton emission computed tomography (SPECT). It works by injecting people with a radioactive substance and then taking images of blood flow in the brain.

SPECT scanning has also been Amen's claim to fame and fortune. In addition to consulting with celebrities beyond the Kardashians, including Justin Bieber, Bella Hadid, and Meghan Trainor, Amen has built a multi-million-dollar empire with a line of BrainMD supplements, television gigs, and even an Amen University offering courses about "brain health and wellness." His chain of Amen Clinics has operated for more than three decades and has seen over 100,000 patients from 155 countries. It was reported in 2012 to be worth $20 million and has since opened six more facilities.

There's nothing wrong with SPECT scanning per se. In fact, it can be a valuable medical tool when it comes to assisting in the diagnosis of structural abnormalities in the brain and body, as well as some neurological conditions. It's also one neuroimaging research tool among many that have invaluably advanced our understanding of the neurobiological contributions to mental disorders, which we know are based in the brain.

But as a clinical psychologist, if someone were to hand me brain images derived from SPECT scanning to help me diagnose a mental disorder, I'd find it as useful as placing my ear against a 50-foot-thick brick wall and trying to hear a patient talk on the other side. Its resolution and clinical utility are that poor.

One outspoken critic of Amen has been fellow psychiatrist Sulman Aziz Mirza. "Amen has pounced on one of psychiatry's greatest criticisms," he told me. "There are no lab tests for depression, no medical imaging for anxiety, no tools in our white coat pockets to measure psychosis. So he's gone ahead and manufactured such a thing for the masses that looks deceptively pretty and scientific but unnecessarily exposes people to radiation for the purpose of prescribing his own line of supplements." The official journal of the American Psychiatric Association would agree with Mirza. After reviewing the evidence, they concluded that neuroimaging of any kind has yet to have a significant impact on the diagnosis or treatment of individual patients in clinical settings.

Patients aren't privy to the science when they visit the Amen Clinics and read its website. "Our database, with over 200,000 brain scans, helps us more successfully identify various types of ADD, anxiety, depression, and many other mental health conditions, so you get the answers you've been looking for," it says. Worse, "We're charging $4000 to tell people they have ADHD and they have to take their supplements," a former employee of the Amen Clinics told The Daily Beast journalist Decca Muldowney in 2023. In her exposé of Amen's grift, Muldowney also spoke with a mother who was not receiving adequate care for her son. "I have not found any value with those brain scans," the mother said, then elaborated, "My overall impression is that although they are offering a human service, a health service, a mental wellness service, that's not their priority. It seems to me that their priority is their business interests."

* * *

Assessment is the bedrock of evidence-based mental health care. If we don't know what's wrong, then we don't know how to help. Legitimate mental health professionals are trained during countless hours of both scholarly and clinical work to understand what contributes to mental health and what leads to mental illness. They're trained to skillfully gather and piece together information from multiple sources using diagnostic interviews, collateral contacts, medical records, and scientifically evaluated test batteries to elucidate the complexity of our mental tapestry. Accurate assessment requires constant collaboration, hypothesis testing, and honesty between mental health professionals and patients to sort out how best to formulate an understanding of a patient's presenting concerns and how to move forward with helpful treatment.

But some get it wrong. In part, that's because trying to understand the mental health and illness of another human being is no easy feat, and as in any area of health care, even our best scientific theories and tools are limited in their capacity to offer accurate and satisfying accounts of our maladies. Other times, however, poor training coupled with poor mental health and science literacy will sour the entire assessment process. The process will turn putrid if one or more of countless pseudoscientific tools are being used to paint wildly inaccurate pictures of a patient's mental life. The online world alone can take us down a rabbit hole of bizarre personality tests (e.g., "What kind of vegetable are you?"), false IQ tests, faulty memory tests, and dangerous Dr. Google self-diagnosis tests, ad nauseam.

Looking to clinical practice, some pseudoscientific assessment tools are so famous or widely used that they're worth telling you about. I have three in mind.

Myers-Briggs Type Indicator. Otherwise known as the MBTI, this tool tries to describe the beautifully colored spectrum of human personality by stripping its vibrancy and force-feeding us with 16 dull personality types. As one random Tumblr user quoted on RationalWiki once said, "The MBTI is a horoscope for nerds." It's a lot more expensive than any horoscope, though. MBTI services make up an industry that rakes in millions per year and is used in both clinical and corporate settings. The psychometric properties of the MBTI—which basically refer to its validity, reliability, and overall legitimacy—are abysmal. It's not good at predicting how you will perform at your job, how well you'll get along with your peers, whether your marriage will end in divorce, the status of your mental health, describing your personality, or really anything else.

Where it is like a horoscope, though, is in how it thrives on the *Barnum effect*, which is one of the thinking errors we learned about in Chapter 6, describing the psychological tendency for people to accept general statements as descriptive of themselves. For example, the vague statement "You have a tendency to be critical of yourself and extraverted at times, but not always," could probably describe both you and me. Similar vague statements are used throughout the MBTI. Well advertised and well funded, it's also overly positive, it avoids describing people negatively, and its results are easily calculated and comprehensible.

Rorschach inkblot. You've likely seen it in movies. It's the test in which a psychologist holds up a series of 10 cards, each containing symmetrical ink splatters, and the patient is told to describe what they see. It's supposed to be a clear and discerning window into the human psyche. It's more like a dirty broken window in an abandoned house from an era long ago. Like the MBTI, its psychometric properties are not up to par. The Rorschach inkblot is a very old test and it's been scientifically scrutinized for well over 50 years. While efforts have been made spanning decades to make it more scientific, it still fails to this day as an evidence-based assessment tool. A charitable reading of the literature lends some validity to its ability to detect perceptual disturbances and disorganized thinking in psychotic disorders such as schizophrenia, but other more valid psychological tests can do that job. It's also unable to help in the assessment of other mental disorders and doesn't do what some of its promoters claim, such as provide a rich and complete picture of a patient's personality or reveal hidden secrets about their emotions or thoughts. A more serious fatal flaw is its well-documented bias to make both adults and children appear psychologically disturbed despite evidence suggesting otherwise. That should cause concern to any clinician who continues to use it—and there are many, unfortunately—particularly in educational, employment, or legal settings where the consequences could be life altering.

Alternative medicine tests. While some chiropractors will suggest that your depression is due to a subluxation in your spine, some naturopathic doctors might say that your body is full of toxins. An acupuncturist may tell you that your life energy is blocked and advise you to see a homeopath, who will prescribe a remedy to balance your vital force, but not before they refer you to a Reiki practitioner to unblock your chakras. The ways in which such alternative medicine practitioners assess for these pseudoscientific "root causes" (a trope from Chapter 5) are as unscientific as they are varied.

For instance, recall that *functional medicine* is one brand of alternative medicine that we learned about in Chapter 4. Science communicator and oncologist David Gorski has described functional medicine as "the worst of both worlds" because "it combines the massive over-testing and over-treatment that can happen in conventional medicine with pure quackery, like 'detoxification,' naturopathy, homeopathy, and chiropractic." At functional medicine clinics, hundreds of expensive laboratory tests are often ordered, many of which are either routine, unnecessary, or bogus. Insidiously, these tests can be used to inform and treat fake diagnoses, such as "adrenal fatigue" or "leaky brain syndrome."

Real Symptoms, Bamboozling Labels

It takes courage and vulnerability to reach out for help when we're struggling with our mental health. Unlike someone with a broken arm, we can't see the source of our suffering. A thorough, well-conducted psychological assessment can aid in our understanding. Sometimes, that assessment will lead to a mental disorder diagnosis that fits and makes sense. Unfortunately, as we discussed in Chapter 3, the science of psychopathology is still evolving, and our current diagnostic categories imperfectly capture aspects of mental illness.

This means at least two things.

First, diagnosis is not the be-all and end-all of assessment and treatment—far from it, in fact. In my own clinical practice, diagnosing mental disorders has been both incredibly useful to patients and, at times, useless. Sometimes, patients are mistakenly referred to our clinic who don't meet diagnostic criteria for any mental disorder. Nevertheless, their pain remains real, and there are still other ways of understanding and helping their mental health concerns.

Second, patients may come to therapy and diagnostically fall through the cracks. For example, a person may exhibit some symptoms from two or more mental disorder categories but too few to meet criteria for any particular diagnosis. An imperfect science of psychopathology necessarily means that we simply don't understand everyone's mental health problems. That gap in our knowledge leaves room not only for frequent misdiagnosis of our suffering among qualified mental health professionals but also for pseudoscientific explanations and exploitation.

In the alternative medicine world, you could be given an entirely fake diagnosis that's not accepted by the broader scientific community. Your symptoms are real! The explanations used to account for your symptoms are not. The malpractice and tragedy of being given a fake diagnosis lies in the misdiagnosis of real, medically unexplained symptoms.

For example, the diagnosis of "adrenal fatigue" is sometimes provided when a patient presents with symptoms that are common to many different conditions, including depression, such as tiredness or low energy and motivation. It was invented by a chiropractor and naturopath named James Wilson, who coined the term in his own book in 1998. The idea behind the diagnosis is that long-term mental or physical stress "drains" the adrenal glands, rendering them unable to produce hormones like cortisol, thereby causing these symptoms. Sometimes people confuse adrenal fatigue with an actual medical condition called adrenal insufficiency that can be diagnosed with laboratory tests and has several causes, such as Addison's disease. The Endocrine Society, representing 18,000 endocrinologists, has stated with respect to adrenal fatigue, "Current medical science recognizes no such condition" and "Doctors are concerned that if you are told you have this condition, the real cause of your symptoms may not be found and treated correctly." As one X (formerly Twitter) user once told me, "When a naturopath diagnosed me with adrenal fatigue, the treatment was to take capsules containing bovine adrenal glands. I asked her to explain how taking ground-up cow gland would heal me and she had no answer. I got the hell out of there."

Another similar example is the lightning rod of a diagnosis called "chronic Lyme disease." There's no debate about the existence of Lyme disease itself, which is the most common tick-borne infection in the northern hemisphere, caused by a bacteria called *Borrelia burgdorferi* and effectively treated with antibiotics. The problem is that the diagnosis of "chronic Lyme disease" is used without clinical evidence of previous Lyme disease to describe patients who experience persistent pain, cognitive dysfunction, fatigue, or all of the above. While the symptoms can be devastating and debilitating, there's no convincing evidence that they're caused by chronic infection or that they can be alleviated with antibiotics or any other number of unsupported and expensive alternative medicine treatments. In a review article published by infectious disease experts in *The New England Journal of Medicine*, they concluded that "chronic Lyme disease" is "not supported by carefully conducted laboratory studies or by controlled treatment trials." They also warn about a community of both practitioners and patients who are convinced of its existence and who "severely criticize" those who challenge its scientific validity, pointing to "the serious harm caused to many patients who have received a misdiagnosis and have been inappropriately treated."

The fake diagnostic merry-go-round continues to sprout new labels, some more scientifically suspect than others. If you've ever seen the hit television series *Better Call Saul*, then you might recognize "electromagnetic hypersensitivity," otherwise known as "Wi-Fi allergies," popularized by the fictional character Chuck McGill. It's an unfortunate, medically disputed diagnosis based on the idea that sensitivity and exposure to low-level electromagnetic fields—from sources such as Wi-Fi, cell phones, computers, and electrical appliances—can cause mental and physical health problems. Some practitioners will sell expensive plastic or metal objects with purported electromagnetic-deflecting powers to "treat" the condition.

Have you heard about "leaky gut syndrome"? You or someone you know may have been duped into believing it's real, a supposed condition in which bacteria and "toxins" are thought to enter the bloodstream through faulty intestinal walls, creating all sorts of havoc from bloating, gas, and cramps to irritability, moodiness, and even autism. The Canadian Society of Intestinal Research calls leaky gut syndrome a myth that's not accepted by mainstream medicine. Riding its coattails is yet another fraudulent diagnosis created by the alternative medicine community to account for all manner of symptoms related to depression, anxiety, fatigue, memory difficulties, and so on. It's called "leaky brain syndrome" (I mentioned it just a few pages ago). In this case, the symptoms are claimed to occur because your brain is degenerating due to "toxins" leaking through a faulty blood–brain barrier. It's a great excuse for practitioners to order costly ill-informed laboratory tests and sell futile dietary supplements.

Indisputable fake diagnoses that defy medical recognition are one thing. Then there's diagnoses that are medically and psychiatrically recognized but still garner much heated controversy. While some withstand the weathering of scientific scrutiny and maintain a spot in the *Diagnostic and Statistical Manual of Mental Disorders*, their existence remains questionable.

The best example is Hollywood's favorite diagnosis: multiple personality disorder, now more formally known as dissociative identity disorder (DID). Think: Robert Louis Stevenson's classic 1885 novel, *The Strange Case of Dr. Jekyll and Mr. Hyde*.

To be diagnosed with DID, a person would need to experience the presence of two or more distinct personalities (called "alters") that recurrently assume control over their behavior. These alters can drastically differ in their personality features from the "host" personality.

You may or may not be surprised to learn that DID does in fact exist insofar as some people do experience different alters. The central controversy is not whether the symptoms of DID exist, but where they come from. There are two major competing theories: One says that alters arise as a consequence of the brain trying to figure out how to deal with horrific childhood abuse; the other says that alters are inadvertently and socially created by clinicians, media influences, and broader cultural expectations and beliefs.

So far, the bulk of scientific literature strongly supports the latter theory, though there are elements of truth to the former as well. As always, it's complicated. And this is why qualified experts are needed to evaluate a person's mental health status with scientifically sound tools. People who experience symptoms consistent with DID find it incredibly distressing, and we don't need pseudoscientific tools and charlatans clouding the picture and adding to that anguish.

Don't Pee on My Mental Health and Tell Me It's Raining

Let's say that a person has undergone an assessment and received an accurate diagnosis to describe their mental health concerns because they navigated their local health care system with finesse and exercised their grift-repellent prowess. Now they need a treatment plan. In part, that will involve dodging a minefield of pseudoscientific treatments where some mines are more clearly visible than others.

One of the biggest take-home messages of this book has been that pseudoscience differs from science in degree rather than in kind, and for that reason, it can be meaningfully identified using the constellation of red flags discussed in Chapter 5. Of those red flags, one carries more weight than others when it comes to separating the wheat from the chaff in mental health care: *absence of connectivity to the broader scientific literature.*

Recall that this warning sign invokes a concept called *scientific plausibility*, which refers to an overall understanding of a scientific question based on existing evidence. In other words, we don't need to start from scratch when considering the likelihood of particular scientific hypotheses or claims—that would be foolish because instead we can draw from the existing mountains of scientific studies that have already been conducted to tell us how plausible those ideas might be. Assessments and treatments that are scientifically implausible are disconnected from hard-earned centuries of biological and medical knowledge. The skeptic community has been shouting from the rooftops about its importance for decades hoping that people will listen. Unfortunately, this message hasn't been well heard among mental health professionals, and it's flagrantly ignored by alternative medicine practitioners. From a patient perspective, it speaks to the importance of using science literacy skills when shopping for care.

Scientific plausibility is the criterion that I'll use going forward in this chapter to differentiate unmistakable cases of pseudoscientific treatments from controversial ones that are more plausible and promising but still plagued with some pseudoscientific features and low-quality evidence to support their use.

Cold Comfort From Hot Air

For her fourth-grade science fair project, a 9-year-old girl named Emily Rosa had a fun idea. She decided to investigate whether therapeutic touch (TT) practitioners could perceive a "human energy field."

Invented by nursing professor Dolores Krieger and clairvoyant Dora Kunz in 1972, TT is described as "energy healing" for anxiety and pain. Its practitioners claim that by passing their hands over a person's body, without making any physical contact, they can detect and manipulate the person's energy field by removing blockages, bringing it into balance, and stimulating the body's natural ability to heal itself.

Rosa's test was simple. She sat down at a table across from practitioners and had them place their arms through a tall, cardboard divider with cutouts at its base, resting their hands, palms up. She then hovered her right hand, palm down, randomly over one of their hands, asking, "Which of your hands do you think my hand is over?" She did this 10 times for each practitioner. Chance alone would produce an average score of 5 out of 10 (50%). After two sets of trials, 21 experienced practitioners responding "left" or "right" repeatedly failed the test and actually performed worse than if they were to flip a coin.

Her fun idea paid off. In 1998, at age 11, she published her findings in the prestigious *JAMA* (*Journal of the American Medical Association*), becoming the youngest person ever published in a peer-reviewed medical journal, and cleanly debunking a central tenet of energy healing along the way.

Case closed, right? Quite the opposite. After reviewing the literature, nursing professor Bernie Garrett showed that TT is still widely promoted internationally. He told me that it remains actively taught in nursing education, and a diagnosis of "imbalanced energy field" appears in the current North American Nursing Diagnosis Association manual. Over five decades of research have failed to support TT or the existence of a human energy field. Nevertheless, a parallel "large body of fabricated and biased bad science has been created to support it," says Garrett. And TT is only one in a long line of "energy medicine" treatments.

Energy medicine. The term "energy medicine" is an umbrella category for the branch of alternative medicine that is sometimes used interchangeably with "energy healing" and "energy psychology." All treatments under this umbrella share the scientifically implausible idea that invisible "human energy fields" are blocked or imbalanced and can be manipulated by practitioners to address mental health and illness. Classic ones include TT, Reiki, polarity therapy, and cranial-sacral therapy. While some use elements of massage and can feel relaxing, you might be better off seeing a registered massage therapist or saving your money and taking a nap.

"Tapping" is one energy medicine technique that's become a sensation. It's been endorsed by entertainers, such as Russell Brand, and amplified on mobile apps, such as The Tapping Solution, developed by motivational speaker Tony Robbins. "After over 1 million plays of our Releasing Anxiety tapping meditation, the average reported reduction of anxiety was 41% in just 9 minutes," claims Robbins's website.

The scientific literature is starkly less enthusiastic. Tapping is what it sounds like: using our fingers to tap various parts of our body along "meridian points" to unblock energy. While meridians are described by alternative medicine practitioners, including acupuncturists, as paths through which our "life-energy" flows, they aren't real anatomical structures, as there's no scientific evidence supporting their existence; the concept of meridians derives from traditional Chinese medicine (TCM), which we'll learn about later. Tapping, unsurprisingly, was inspired by an acupuncture class taken by psychologist Roger Callahan, who went on to develop a treatment called thought field therapy (TFT) in 1997 after instructing a patient to firmly tap the area under her eye to hit invisible energy fields called "thought fields," leading to a miraculous recovery from her severe phobia of water.

TFT then spawned several offshoot therapies, the most popular being emotional freedom techniques (EFT), developed by Gary Craig, who studied under Callahan. The main difference is that TFT asks patients to use a variety of tapping procedures to treat several psychological problems, whereas EFT uses one simplified tapping procedure to address everything from autism to warts.

What's deceptively irksome about promoters of both TFT and EFT is that they'll tell you their treatments "work" but won't tell you the real reasons that they could *appear* to work. In addition to invoking placebo effects and factors common to all talk therapies, these treatments also incorporate carelessly applied ideas derived from cognitive-behavioral therapy, a well-established treatment. This means that any pseudoscientific studies used in marketing materials showing they "work" can easily be explained by factors other than their implausible theoretical underpinnings.

Naturopathy. "I left naturopathy with a bang," confesses Britt Marie Hermes, a former naturopathic doctor and graduate from one of the most influential schools of naturopathy in North America, Bastyr University, on her website. She continues: "Naturopathy is not what I was led to believe. The profession functions as a system of indoctrination based on discredited ideas about health and medicine, full of pseudoscientific rhetoric and loaded with ineffective and dangerous practices." Since abandoning ship, Hermes has been on a mission to expose the ethical and scientific duplicity of alternative medicine practitioners despite facing tremendous personal and legal hostility. For her efforts, she was awarded the John Maddox Prize in 2018, which is administered by the science communication organization Sense About Science in partnership with the top medical journal *Nature* to individuals who promote sound science in the face of hardship.

According to the Canadian Association of Naturopathic Doctors, naturopathy is an umbrella term encompassing "diet and lifestyle changes, natural therapies including botanical medicine, clinical nutrition, hydrotherapy, homeopathy, naturopathic manipulation and traditional Chinese medicine/acupuncture." It's described as "a distinct primary health care system that blends modern scientific knowledge with traditional and natural forms of medicine," and its "philosophy is to stimulate the healing power of the body and treat the underlying causes of disease."

If you've read Chapters 5 and 6, then you might be able to swiftly recognize the fallacies (i.e., *appeal to tradition*, *appeal to nature*) and alternative medicine trope (i.e., *addressing the root cause*) inherent to their definition.

Problematically, the way in which naturopathic doctors treat the underlying cause of mental health concerns is dependent on the often-implausible theoretical rationale for the particular treatments used.

For example, if you want to improve your depression or personal relationships, then a homeopath might offer you some Berlin Wall pills to "break down your emotional barriers." While that specific example might seem rare and strange, it's no stranger than one of the principles on which all homeopathic remedies are premised: namely, the "law of minimum dose," which we discussed in Chapter 5. Recall that in practical terms, it means that all homeopathic remedies are so diluted that no molecules of the original substance remain, leading to the absurd upshot that your recommended Berlin Wall pills wouldn't even contain actual fragments of the Berlin Wall. Instead, they should just contain water and its "memory." Disastrously, due to such a poorly regulated homeopathy industry, many remedies are in fact mislabeled and contain potentially harmful ingredients.

Hermes told me that when she attended Bastyr University, she was required to take three quarters of homeopathy to graduate, and only one quarter of pharmacology, noting that homeopathy is an integral part of naturopathic practice. When she went back to her student notebook, she found a number of homeopathic treatments for depression, including *Aurum metallicum*, which she said is the remedy of choice for patients experiencing suicidal thoughts. "I distinctly remember being told in homeopathy class that if a patient is showing signs of harming themselves, give Aurum first, and *then* assess for safety," she told me.

Like a homeopath, an acupuncturist may wish to treat your alcohol addiction by inserting thin needles into the "meridian points" on your body to relieve blockages in the flow of a "life-energy" source called "Qi" or "Chi," ignoring the unconvincing evidence base. They may also wish to give you an herbal product sourced from TCM, assuring you that their remedy has evolved over thousands of years, to restore your balance of two opposing energies in the universe: Yin (representing all things that are *motionless, cold, downward, inner, inhibitory*, etc.) and Yang (representing *active, hot, upward, outside, stimulatory*, etc.). The TCM approach is tightly related to ancient Chinese philosophy, banking on concepts such as Qi, Chi, Yin, and Yang to inform a variety of treatments such as acupuncture, herbal medicine, and other kinds of mind–body practices like cupping therapy, tai chi, and qigong. Notwithstanding TCM's scientifically unsubstantiated theories about the flow of energies and their impact on mental health, some Chinese herbal

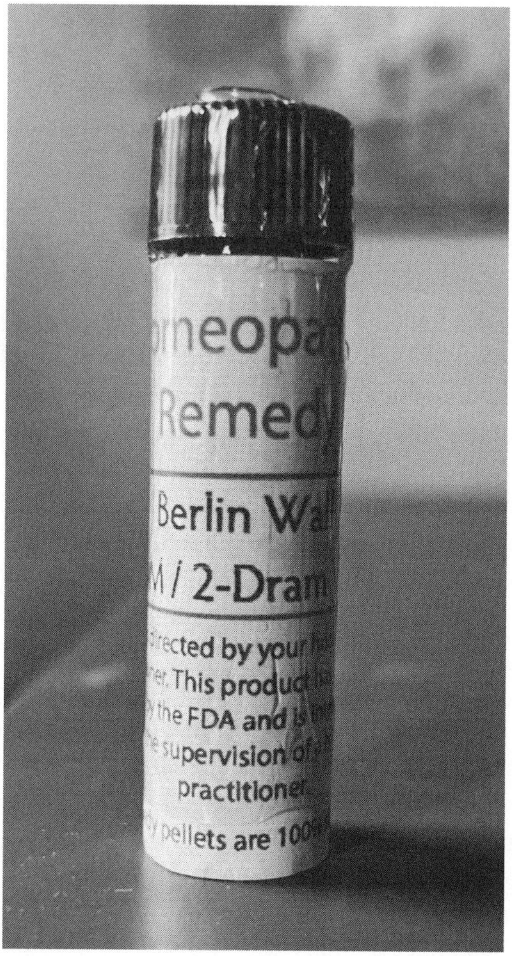

Homeopathic Berlin Wall pills to "break down your emotional barriers."

products have been found to be contaminated with undeclared plant and animal materials, drugs, heavy metals, and pesticides, some of which have been known to cause organ damage.

Or a naturopathic doctor may reach into their toolkit and draw from orthomolecular medicine, which was popularized by Linus Pauling, who won a Nobel Prize in Chemistry in 1954 and who later became widely criticized as suffering from Nobel disease (see Chapter 6) for arguing that megadoses of vitamin C could effectively treat schizophrenia. Nowadays, "orthomolecular psychiatry" is a fringe ideology that hyperfocuses on the role of poor nutrition as "the root cause" of mental illness and therefore uses dietary supplements as treatment despite rejection by evidence-based mental health care. All of these "root causes" are scientifically untenable.

Ayurveda. Criticizing the scientific integrity of Ayurveda could get me in trouble, given its ties to the government of India's Ministry of AYUSH (Ayurveda, Unani, Siddha, and Homeopathy) and entrenchment in Indian culture. But even the alternative medicine–friendly National Center for Complementary and Integrative Health (NCCIH)—the lead agency for alternative medicine research in the U.S. government—acknowledges that "there is little scientific evidence on Ayurveda's value for other health issues" beyond a few "small or not well-designed" studies on pain, osteoarthritis, and type 2 diabetes.

Ayurveda is a prescientific, belief-based Indian medical system founded on ancient writings that rely on a "natural" and "holistic" approach to physical and mental health. It combines lifestyle recommendations with products derived from plants, animals, metals, and minerals. The NCCIH warns that Ayurvedic preparations can contain lead, mercury, or arsenic in amounts that could be toxic.

This tracks with the clinical experience of India-based hepatologist and physician-scientist Cyriac Abby Phillips, who, like Hermes, has been facing intense personal and legal backlash since 2017 for being a well-known whistleblower. "The old-school belief that Ayurveda is herbal, natural, and safe is deeply ingrained into the minds of the people here, but this isn't so—my research group's seminal and disruptive work proved that Ayurvedic herbal drugs threatened public health, causing severe liver injuries in many, while some patients died," he told me.

Those safety concerns are worrisome beyond India. With celebrities like Kourtney Kardashian and Gwyneth Paltrow selling products linked to Ayurveda on their respective wellness sites, Poosh and Goop, at least one research firm has estimated the global Ayurveda market could grow to $6.8 billion by 2026.

When I spoke with Phillips, he described how Ayurvedic texts detail in depth their own unfounded claims about the assessment and treatment of mental disorders. Scientifically obsolete theories are still taught in Ayurveda colleges, such as the humor theory of Ayurveda, which seeks balance between Kapha (phlegm), Vata (air/space), and Pitta (bile). "For instance, Ayurveda teaches that the treatment of *unmada* (mania) includes bloodletting, purgation, enemas, and induced vomiting," he told me.

As we discussed in Chapter 4, one crucial challenge of evidence-based mental health care is respecting and incorporating different belief systems in culturally competent ways while sidestepping harm, pseudoscience, and practices that are misappropriated by the wellness industry. It's also true that there remains an enduring need to question the science behind particular practices that may carry cultural value but are at odds with modern medicine and risk derailing competent patient care, no matter the potential to offend critics.

Chiropractic. Millions of people in North America spend billions of dollars each year visiting chiropractors to hear their spines "pop." Few realize that chiropractic is rooted in mystical ideas. Its birthday is said to be September 18, 1895, when Daniel David Palmer "adjusted" the spine of a janitor named Harvey Lillard, allegedly curing his deafness. Convincing himself that 95% of all diseases—such as "insanity, sexual dysfunction, measles, and influenza"—were caused by displaced vertebrae, Palmer went on to open chiropractic schools and even seriously considered establishing chiropractic as a religion. He coined the term "innate intelligence" to describe the "energy" or "vital force" that enables the body to heal itself. Chiropractors manipulate the spine to correct vertebral "subluxations" that block the flow of the "innate."

The confusing part is that "subluxation" is a common medical term. Real orthopedic subluxations are partial dislocations between joint surfaces. They exist and show up on x-rays, whereas chiropractic subluxations don't: They're undetectable and there's no science to support their existence. Not all modern chiropractors buy into imaginary subluxations, but many do, and they market the scientifically implausible idea to patients.

Colleagues of mine conducted an analysis of chiropractic clinic websites in my home province of Alberta, Canada. Out of 121 websites, one-third presented a theory of chiropractic subluxation relating to a vast range of health issues, including attention-deficit hyperactivity disorder (ADHD), autism, prostate cancer, multiple sclerosis, Parkinson's disease, pregnancy and fetus development, stomach problems, and hormonal imbalances—some websites included such marketing for newborns, infants, and children.

Equally concerning is that, if you Google your own local chiropractic clinics, you will find some that claim to be able to help with a broad range of mental health concerns such as anxiety, depression, addiction, and even learning disorders. Some chiropractors do great work when it comes to treating low back pain with spinal manipulation therapy, which also happens to be used in other professions, such as physiotherapy. Beyond back pain, however, the science doesn't support the use of spinal manipulation therapy for anything else, including mental disorders.

Dishonorable mentions. As we've been surveying these broad categories of energy medicine, naturopathy, Ayurveda, and chiropractic, you might've noticed one common thread weaved throughout all of them: It's called *vitalism*.

The "human energy field" in TT, the "thought fields" in TFT, the "vital force" in homeopathy, the "Qi or Chi" in acupuncture and TCM, "prana" in Ayurveda, "innate intelligence" in chiropractic, and so on—all these terms describe a kind of magical life-giving energy force that cannot be scientifically measured. Vitalism refers to the belief that living things are different from nonliving things because they possess this life-force energy that exists outside the laws of physics and chemistry. Ironically, alternative medicine practitioners who promote treatments rooted in vitalism pretend to be scientific anyway, sometimes drawing from pseudoscientific journals to sell their claims.

While vitalism lies at the underbelly of many popular alternative medicine treatments, it's not the only unscientific belief floating around mental health care. Some treatments are uniquely implausible in their own right with no evidence to support their use and despite ubiquitous marketing to the contrary. This book can't possibly expose them all, but I've listed some more that are worth knowing about in addition to the ones covered under the heading "Unequivocal Pseudoscientific Treatments" on pages 211–213 in "Mind the Takeaways."

Entering Hotly Contested Zones

Ever since I started full-time clinical work, I've felt the tension inherent to practicing clinical psychology from an evidence-based perspective. People come to therapy wanting relief, and when they don't experience it from established treatments, they look to alternatives. It's easy to explain the implausibility and lack of science behind unequivocal pseudoscientific treatments when someone asks for my opinion. It's much more difficult in the pseudoscience gray zone, where treatments may hold promise but there's a gap between the hype about those treatments and the research supporting the hype.

In these cases, there may be a few red flags that irritate our spidey senses, but the approaches are worth exploring and may one day accumulate enough evidence to cross the somewhat arbitrary boundary into the realm of evidence-based care. For now, though, and for good reasons, they aren't yet ready for prime time. In surveying these approaches, our science and mental health literacy skills are really put to the test.

Cannabis. For more than a decade I've been involved in cannabis research and education. When I wrote a couple articles in *Scientific American* about the most up-to-date science on the relationship between cannabis and mental health, I purchased a front-row seat to the cannabis culture wars between pro- and anti-cannabis zealots, and I received vitriol from both factions. So I wrote about that too, highlighting that the war is futile because cannabis itself is so complex that it's better understood not as a single substance, but as a chemical soup with over 500 ingredients that can be served in an untold number of ways.

The two most studied of these ingredients are THC (delta-9-tetrahydrocannabinol) and CBD (cannabidiol), which have very different effects on a person's experience. For example, THC can induce euphoria, anxiety, and psychosis, whereas CBD is largely nonintoxicating and can produce anti-anxiety and anti-psychotic effects. If you scour the scientific literature, you'll find evidence that cannabis could have benefits for a variety of conditions, ranging from nausea, epilepsy, and multiple sclerosis to opioid withdrawal and social anxiety disorder. It's also linked to harms, including addiction, anxiety, psychosis, cardiovascular disease, and cognitive impairment. Nothing about cannabis is straightforward, and its use in mental health care needs to be approached with nuance and a critical eye, especially when considering its role in a person's life and treatment plan.

Psychedelics. Everything old is new again. It's not uncommon for patients to ask me whether they should try "microdosing" psilocybin—that is, taking a very small amount of the active ingredient in magic mushrooms—to help treat their depression. And why wouldn't they ask? They've read in the media about new studies showing that psilocybin can cure depression and PTSD, that ketamine can too, or that microdosing LSD (also known as "acid") can make someone more creative. These are tough conversations.

The enthusiasm for psychedelics in mental health care dates to at least the 1960s when at that time, pioneers of psychedelic research, such as the psychologist Timothy Leary, were conducting preliminary work on LSD and psilocybin. Such research was essentially shut down until recently due to government legislation and regulation of controlled substances. In the last decade or so, psychedelic research and popularity have been revived amid the desire to improve mental health care, commercial interests, and changing societal attitudes.

In 2022, my own University of Calgary established a $3 million research position, headed by behavioral neuroscientist Leah Mayo, dedicated to investigating the therapeutic potential of psychedelics. What's more, in 2023 Alberta became the first Canadian province to regulate psychedelic therapies for mental disorders, meaning that patients are now legally allowed to receive psychedelic treatment under the supervision of a psychiatrist.

Unfortunately, psychedelic research is notorious for being plagued with bad science—such as drawing conclusions based on small sample sizes, as well as lack of blinding and high dropout rates in randomized controlled trials—but the situation is improving. The majority of research has focused on the use of psilocybin and ketamine for anxiety, depression, PTSD, and addiction, although other hallucinogens such as MDMA (also known as "ecstasy"), LSD, peyote, ibogaine, and ayahuasca have been explored. While the exact ways in which these substances work vary, they all impact mood and behavior and can produce a variety of effects, including euphoria, hallucinations, changes in perception, and spiritual experiences.

In terms of the evidence base, psilocybin and ketamine have received the most support in their ability to improve mental health concerns. But the science isn't great and contains mixed results, including the potential for adverse effects like headache, nausea, dizziness, and suicidal thoughts.

Trying to self-medicate symptoms away without the assistance of a professional could be an issue too. One study showed that 33% of people who said they had a diagnosis of bipolar disorder described new or worsening symptoms of mania, sleep problems, and anxiety after psilocybin trips.

It's also important to know that many studies are investigating the use of "psychedelic-assisted therapy," which means that they're looking at using psychedelics together with psychotherapy over the course of several months (e.g., the administration of MDMA during three psychotherapy sessions out of a total of 15 psychotherapy sessions). This means that evidence found for "psychedelic-assisted therapy" doesn't mean that psychedelics are quick fixes or that they work by themselves. The field is still very much in its infancy.

Twelve-step programs. Nearly every business day for more than 10 years, I've been driving to my local hospital to help people who experience the carnage of addiction. Together, we participate in individual therapy, group therapy, medication reviews, and other appointments relevant to their treatment plan. Outside of our clinic, patients are encouraged to enlist the help of other resources too. Very often, these resources involve getting help from peers who are going through the same challenges. Among the most popular kinds of peer support groups are 12-step programs, such as Alcoholics Anonymous (AA), Narcotics Anonymous (NA), and Gamblers Anonymous (GA).

Since their creation in the 1930s by cofounders Bill Wilson and Bob Smith, 12-step programs have been controversial in the addiction community and the general public. As the name implies, all 12-step programs are based on walking through the 12 steps detailed in *Alcoholics Anonymous*, the 1939 publication colloquially referred to as the "Big Book." Wilson and Smith's philosophy takes a hard stance on the nature of addiction, viewing it as a lifelong disease that requires complete abstinence for recovery. Many alcohol and drug treatment programs throughout North America are based on 12-step principles and mandate abstinence from their participants.

From a scientific perspective, the evidence for 12-step programs is as mixed as it is tangled. Since there are so many of them offered in the community without oversight, a 12-step group held online may differ vastly in terms of content and quality than the one offered in the church down the road. Perhaps counter to what some may think, some of the more formally structured ones do have a solid body of evidence supporting their use. The benefits of 12-step programs can largely be explained by the power of the group: We feel healthier when we feel heard and socially connected rather than carrying the monstrous burden of addiction alone. Our chances of benefiting from such groups increase when we experience this connection.

Twelve-step programs can become problematic when they undermine other evidence-based treatments. For example, the strict, abstinence-only philosophy of 12-step programs may prohibit the use of psychiatric medications. Many of my patients who experience opioid addiction or ADHD have been told they're not welcome in some programs because they use opioid agonist therapies (OATs) and stimulant medications, which are first-line, medically recommended treatments, despite the fact that other substances like caffeine and nicotine may be allowed. These are arbitrary boundaries.

The scientific literature has also left behind aspects of the outdated 12-step philosophy itself. Not everyone who experiences an addiction requires complete abstinence to recover. In situations where an abstinence-based policy is rigidly enforced, attending 12-step programs may harm more than they help.

Hypnosis. For some people, the word *hypnosis* dredges up images of audience members involuntarily clucking around like chickens on a stage at the whim of a hypnotist with a pocket watch. These depictions reflect the myth that hypnosis causes an altered state of consciousness prompting participants to lose all control. Stage hypnosis is entertainment. It's been well explained by factors such as the willingness to please, individual differences in suggestibility (i.e., the tendency to act on the suggestions of others), outright trickery, and straightforward invitations to play along with the show.

Real hypnosis, or hypnotherapy, involves the induction of a deeply relaxed state—sometimes called a *hypnotic trance*—during which a person is instructed to imagine changes in sensations, perceptions, memories, thoughts, emotions, and behaviors. After a hypnotic induction, those who do happen to experience these changes are more likely to expect them, be motivated to have them, and be suggestible. We can see the hypnotic trance in the brain too: Neuroimaging studies have shown that hypnosis involves changes in certain brain regions, such as those related to self-awareness and attention. While that might sound spectacular, the findings are unsurprising. They're exactly what we would expect to see following the induction of a deeply relaxed state where one feels more absorbed and focused than usual.

Hypnosis has enjoyed a long history as a controversial treatment for mental disorders, dating back to its 18th-century roots when physician Franz Anton Mesmer was "mesmerizing" participants and some scholars were claiming that hypnosis allowed people to astral travel, see through skin without the use of eyes, and experience paranormal phenomena. Centuries later, hypnosis is no longer best understood as an altered state of consciousness, and there's an accumulating body of research showing that it could be helpful in treating some conditions, such as pain and tobacco addiction, though it's still up for debate whether these benefits occur for reasons beyond relaxation, placebo effects, and other factors common to talk therapies that are associated with hypnosis.

Today, hypnosis can be hijacked by practitioners and implemented as a method in pseudoscientific treatments such as past life regression therapy as if it were still capable of extraordinary powers. With no shortage of wellness websites asserting extravagant claims—like hypnosis is "30 times more effective for weight loss" compared with no treatment—we need to remain wary of the way hypnosis is packaged and sold.

Practitioners may try to impress you with their certifications, but anyone can practice hypnotherapy without being a licensed mental health professional. In 2009, even an orange and white tabby cat named George became registered as a hypnotherapist in the United Kingdom. George's owner, Chris Jackson, presenter of the BBC show *Inside Out*, teasingly demonstrated the weakness of the certification process by registering him with the United Fellowship of Hypnotherapists, the Professional Hypnotherapy Practitioner Association, and the British Board of Neuro Linguistic Programming.

Mindfulness meditation. In 2004, Andy Puddicombe returned to the United Kingdom from a 10-year expedition training as a Buddhist monk. He set up his own private meditation practice and cofounded with Richard Pierson a company that owns the mindfulness meditation mobile app *Headspace*, currently valued at $3 billion. Its rival app, *Calm*, is valued at $2 billion. I suppose we can give credit to the wellness industry for monetizing philosophies that eschew material possessions.

Mindfulness is everywhere. It's built into the fabric of the wellness community. It's in schools, workplaces, and hospitals. It's even offered in my own clinic and was the subject of my very first scientific publication as an undergraduate student. And yet, many people don't understand what it is, partly because it's a tricky concept and partly because what's often called mindfulness can look different depending on who's facilitating its classes.

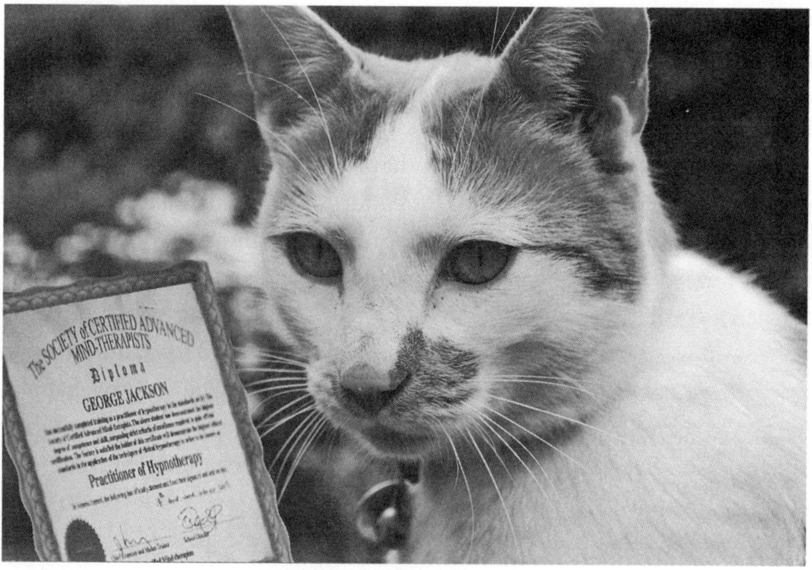

George the cat, registered hypnotherapist.
Image credit: Chris Jackson

It's also an umbrella term. Mindfulness is used to describe numerous practices and theoretical concepts related to attention, awareness, memory, and acceptance. It's commonly summarized as a mantra of cultivating attention toward our experiences by observing them in the present moment without judgment. The term has its historical footing in Buddhism and was first transformed into a treatment approach by Jon Kabat-Zinn, who developed "mindfulness-based stress reduction" for pain. Mindfulness then became adapted by researchers and incorporated into other treatment protocols, notably ones that carry scientific evidence to support their use, such as "mindfulness-based relapse prevention" for addiction, "mindfulness-based cognitive therapy" for depression, and as an important component in the evidence-based treatments of dialectical behavior therapy (DBT) and acceptance and commitment therapy (ACT).

The ubiquity of mindfulness, however, doesn't live up to its hype. You may be disappointed to learn that mindfulness research has been heavily criticized by scholars for its poor quality, with lax methods and ill-defined concepts—so poor, in fact, that the shortcomings of mindfulness research hamper our ability to draw meaningful conclusions from its many positive findings. To make things worse, newer research is starting to show that mindfulness can cause harm. For instance, one recent review of 83 studies found that the most common negative experiences with mindfulness included increases in anxiety, depression, disorientation, confusion, attention/memory problems, perceptual hypersensitivity, stress, and hallucinations. Mindfulness may be seen as a panacea, but it's an illusory one propped up by flimsy science and lavishly oversold claims.

Purple hat therapies. Pretend you have a splitting headache. You've run out of ibuprofen and are feeling so desperate for pain relief that you ask your friendly neighbor if they have any. They regrettably don't but offer to pop by to help. They describe themself as a wellness coach and tell you they've just learned a revolutionary new treatment for pain called "purple hat therapy." They say it was recently tested in a randomized controlled trial and shown to work. So you oblige. When they come over, they hand you a purple hat and tell you to wear it because it has healing properties. You're then instructed to take a pill, do five jumping jacks, do 10 burpees, and chant the phrase "I am one with the universe" three times. You think it sounds silly, but you do it anyway. Twenty minutes later, your headache starts to dissipate.

Was it the purple hat? The pill? The particular combination of jumping jacks, burpees, and chants? Unbeknownst to you and them, the pill contained ibuprofen and that's why you feel better. The rest of the bells and whistles did nothing to contribute to your relief. The developers of purple hat therapy claim that while the pill may have been partly helpful, it's the other components of the therapy that matter.

Purple hat therapy is a fictional metaphor. It was an argument used in 2003 by psychologists Gerald Rosen and Gerald Davison to critique the way we define evidence-based treatments that lack scientific plausibility—and more specifically, to critique the up-and-coming revolutionary new treatment at the time, eye movement desensitization and reprocessing therapy (EMDR).

Originally developed in the 1980s by Francine Shapiro to target PTSD symptoms, EMDR is a treatment involving a practitioner leading a patient through a sequence of eye movements while they are thinking about the most salient parts of a traumatic memory. This act of thinking about the memory is a highly effective strategy called imaginal exposure that is also used in cognitive-behavioral therapy (CBT). Rosen and Davison argued that in EMDR, the eye movements were a purple hat.

More than 20 years later, EMDR has established itself as an evidence-based treatment for PTSD, but the necessity of the eye movement component remains controversial. Overall, the bulk of evidence from clinical trials doesn't support the idea that eye movements are a critical component of treatment.

To many mental health professionals, this news sounds unnerving, especially in light of endorsements from bestselling books, such as *The Body Keeps the Score*; offshoot panacea-like therapies that utilize eye movements, such as accelerated resolution therapy; and an entire industry that sells kits, wands, and pulsating lightbars meant to facilitate eye movements.

Using our science literacy skills is key when thinking about what other treatments might in essence be purple hat therapies. Are the tapping procedures in EFT purple hats? When paired with relaxing music, are the patterned beats in biosound therapy purple hats? What about acupuncture needles? Are cranial-sacral therapists really balancing our energy fields or do we just relish a good head massage?

Animal-assisted therapies. When I told a trusted friend that I'd be writing about animal-assisted therapies in the context of pseudoscience, they asked, "What kind of monster are you? Who doesn't love puppies?" I had to correct them. Animal-assisted therapies don't refer to having pets or service animals or emotional support animals. Those aren't treatments. They refer to a variety of therapy approaches marketed as a fun and calming way to treat mental disorders, such as equine-assisted therapy, dolphin-assisted therapy, and wolf-assisted therapy. Even baby goat yoga has been touted to benefit mental disorders—and of course having your own personal goat to frolic around with during yoga would bring laughter and joy to almost anyone.

But let's resist trivializing the severity of mental disorders. The science shows that all animal-assisted therapies have at least two, if not three, similar problems. First, they're typically claimed to work in scientifically implausible ways, such as dolphins sending "healing energy" through ultrasound or horses being able to "balance internal feelings and banish negative emotions." Second, the research literature supporting their use is peppered with serious flaws related to study design, rendering results nearly impossible to interpret. And third, in cases involving wild animals, ethical concerns have been raised from the standpoint of captive animal welfare and disease spread.

All things considered, using animals could be helpful to facilitate mental health strategies that we know work, such as engaging in activities that are effortful and pleasurable. Patients can even develop strong therapeutic relationships with their animal-assisted therapists. But these benefits could also be achieved in other ways without resorting to such expensive and theoretically flawed means.

* * *

When we hear pseudo-profound bullshit from a scientist, we're more likely to believe it than when we hear the exact same bullshit from a spiritual guru. That's what researchers publishing in *Nature* found when they presented people with computer-generated meaningless statements that were attributed to either a scientist or guru. They dubbed their finding the *Einstein effect.*

When credible scientists and health professionals like Brian L. Weiss and Daniel G. Amen speak gobbledygook about assessment and treatment, they capitalize on the Einstein effect, and we're likely to listen to them. This kind of credential misuse only begins to scratch the surface of the mountainous wellness industry that cheats its way into our heads.

It's wise to remain leery of anything touted as a "miracle cure" or "breakthrough." The scientific community owes it to people who experience mental health concerns to exhaust every possible avenue of plausible treatments. But from an evidence-based perspective that values competence, safety, and ethics, it needs to be done right and in a way that doesn't put the cart before the horse.

Alternative medicine lights the cart on fire before the horse even arrives on scene. With no principled compass guiding its growth, grifters are allowed to con, and pseudoscience flourishes unchecked. In contempt of alternative medicine supposedly living at the margins of mainstream medicine, it has firmly set up shop in mental health care and isn't going anywhere—in fact, it's metastasizing.

If you're thinking to yourself, "Gosh, so far this book sounds pretty dismal," I agree. Let me now show you solutions.

PART 3
GOOD SCIENCE

8

What Mental Health Really Means

Many people are familiar with Andrew Tate. He came to my attention during a recent night out when a friend voiced her concern about the attitude of her 16-year-old son. For the past year, he was becoming increasingly distant from his parents and extremely snappy. It was nothing too out of the ordinary for a teenager, until he started watching videos online of Andrew Tate's self-anointed pearls of wisdom. "Have you heard of this Tate guy, Jonathan?" my friend asked. Admittedly, I hadn't. So, she showed me some of his tweets:

- Depression isn't real. You feel sad, you move on. You will always be depressed if your life is depressing. Change it. Thread.
- There are very few fat lonely man, aged 60. With no money or family or hobbys. Who arnt depressed. — this is not a clinical disease.
- It is a circumstance which they must change. Most "depressed" people are unhappy with their lives, too lazy to change it. That simple.
- Then they pretend they caught some disease to absolve all responsibility. ITS NOT MY FAULT IM SAD. Yes it is.
- So people defend depression. They get angry when I say this. Because they need this bullshit to justify their own failures.

"How can my son believe the crap this guy is saying, let alone like him?" my exasperated friend wondered. I empathized with her as she continued. "He knows severe depression runs in our family and last night he called us whiny bitches for having therapists. What if he becomes depressed? What do I do?" I had no easy answers for her. As a friend, I could only lend a trusted ear and point to resources for both him and her if she felt they were needed. Part of me wanted to downplay Tate's influence, but I couldn't.

In 2022, NBC News ran a story about him entitled "The Internet Can't Stop Talking About Andrew Tate." Self-described as a "success coach," Tate is a social media influencer and former championship-winning kickboxer. His misogynistic content is banned from Facebook, YouTube, Instagram, and TikTok, but that hasn't stopped his reach. As of August 2022, the TikTok hashtag #AndrewTate had been viewed 12.7 billion times. While he was banned from X (formerly Twitter), he was reinstated following Elon Musk's takeover and currently boasts over 7 million followers. He's been accused of running a social media pyramid scheme via a subscription-based online course called Hustler's University 2.0, as well as involvement in a Romanian human trafficking ring (although he denies all claims of wrongdoing). Consistent with my friend's experience, ABC News (Australia) reported the results of a survey that interviewed more than 500 teenage boys across 24 schools, finding that 28% said they looked up to Andrew Tate. "He's a top G, he's a cool guy, he knows what he's doing," said one participant.

It's hard to pick just one problem associated with Tate's clout. The acceptance of his inaccurate and stigmatizing view about mental health is only one damaging piece of his persona, but it's emblematic of an unnerving trend that lurks at the core of today's culture. The author Tom Nichols named it "the death of expertise," to describe the phenomenon where uninformed opinions have increasingly come to carry the same weight as expert ones. The term *armchair quarterback* refers to an angry football fan who shouts at the TV while watching at home, but it's adaptable to anyone who acts like they have all the answers to a problem without any experience or qualifications. Andrew Tate is among the loudest armchair psychologists on the internet. It pains me to say this, but the field of psychology itself is partly to blame.

Up until now, this book has heavily focused on critiquing the pseudoscience derived from alternative medicine and the wellness industry. "Jonathan, you know you're a psychologist, right?" is a snarky question that I often get asked incredulously by people who troll my social media accounts. "Look in the mirror! Why don't you clean your own house? You're soft, Jonathan, just like psychology because it's a pseudoscience." These comments are meant to offend me. But I have to laugh, not because I enjoy being insulted, but because I agree with some of the sentiments. We need to strengthen psychology's scientific chops.

Psychology has a public relations problem, and owning up to it has been a long time coming. In 2008, the American Psychological Association conducted a large survey sampling the public's attitudes about psychology. It found that only 30% of participants viewed psychology as scientific and that 41% believed it's less rigorous than medical research. In a *Los Angeles Times* opinion piece, journalist Alex B. Berezow concluded in 2012 that "Psychology isn't a science," igniting a firestorm of moans and pushback from my fellow psychologists. Then it got worse.

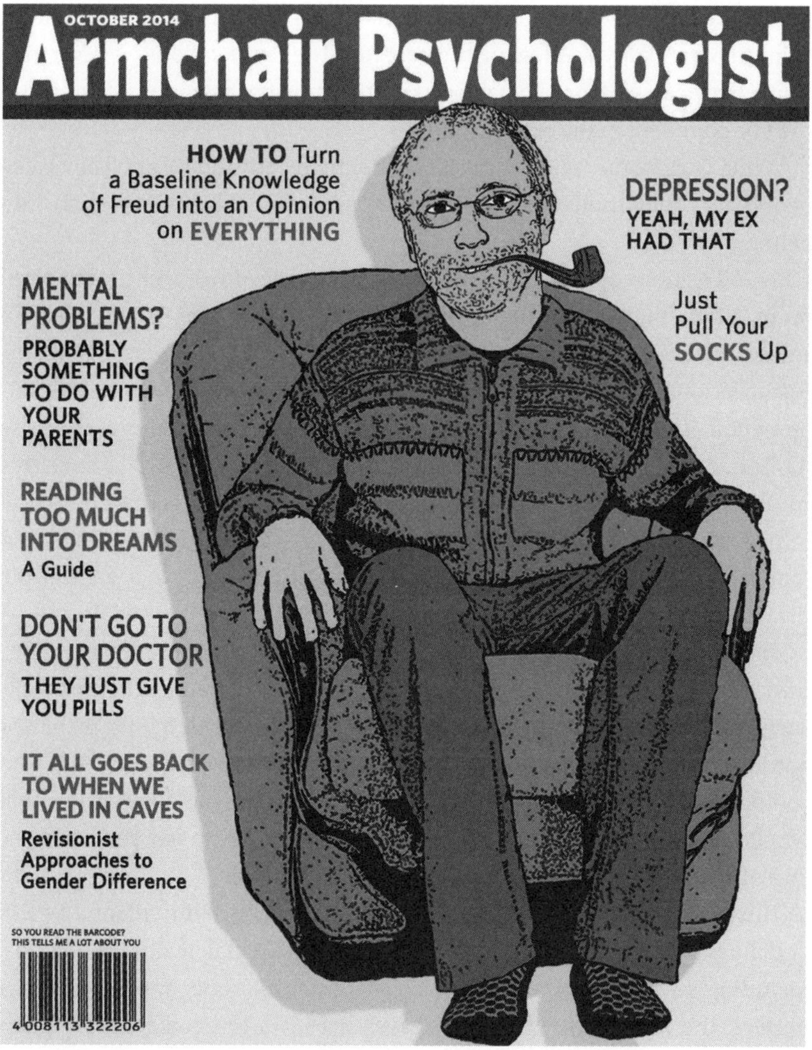

Copyright Mustard The Comedy Mag, Words: Andrew O'Neill, Illustration: Skinny Gaviar. http://www.mustardweb.org/moviesmags/armchairpsychologist.htm

The 2010s were marked by something academics called psychology's *replication crisis*, though it also applied to areas of medicine. It meant that when scientists tried to replicate prior research with new participants and tighter methods, many previous classic and highly cited studies demonstrated weaker effects or failed to replicate entirely. Some subdisciplines, such as personality psychology, fared better than others, such as social psychology. Clinical psychology was feeling the heat too. The ramifications were very serious: How can we learn to balance skepticism with trust in expertise if we can't be confident in the expertise?

While worrisome, scientific crises are actually advantageous. They wake people up. They motivate scientists to learn from their mistakes and do better.

In 2023, more optimistic news arrived. A team of researchers analyzed more than 14,000 psychology studies since the year 2000. Certain subdisciplines had higher likelihoods of replicating, such as personality, organizational, and clinical, compared to cognitive, social, and developmental. The studies conducted by researchers who had more expertise replicated better, and studies featured in the media replicated worse. This speaks to the idea that the news is not a good place to get your psychological information. Overall, the team concluded that studies showed improved replicability from 2010 to 2019, suggesting that scientists have been heeding the call.

The truth is that psychology is a mixed bag. Some areas are clearly scientific, while others are less so; still others are floridly pseudoscientific. This isn't unique to psychology, but that doesn't excuse its desperate need for hardier scientific footing. We need to remain just as wary of claims from psychology as we do of those from alternative medicine. The difference is that psychology is philosophically willing to grow and works to self-correct in the face of error, typifying the heart of a scientific discipline.

The domain of clinical psychology deals with improving mental health and illness. It's joined in its efforts by other allied mental health professions, including psychiatry. Their approach is a scientific one, and though imperfect, the knowledge they offer saves lives. As the comedian Stephen Fry once remarked, "Of course science doesn't know everything. But because science doesn't know everything, that doesn't mean science knows nothing."

In this chapter, we'll talk about the concepts that inform evidence-based mental health care, including what makes good therapy. We'll survey ways to improve mental health and illness that are backed by science, while keeping our eyes open to the sobering limitations of our knowledge. Whereas grifters will promise you the world and tell you what you want to hear, honest mental health professionals will join you in a frank discussion about what we know and what we don't.

Evidence-Based What?

For over a decade I've provided supervision to students in clinical psychology, social work, nursing, and medicine. "I'm here to learn how to do therapy" is what almost all of them announce on their first day at my clinic. Teaching them is a tall order—because I'm *still* learning how to do therapy. After thousands of hours of clinical training and experience as a graduate student outside the classroom and research lab, I often tell students that it wasn't until I became fully licensed and started working that my real learning began. An appeal to lifelong learning might sound like a cliché, but it's deeper than that for mental health care professionals who are bound to the philosophy of evidence-based practice. Let's step back in time for a moment to explain what I mean.

Recall from Chapter 4 that the Flexner Report of 1910 ushered in modern medicine by emphasizing that science should be at the center of health care. It took a while, but eventually the discipline of clinical psychology came to the same conclusion. Its renaissance occurred in 1947 when the American Psychological Association decided that clinical psychology should adopt the integration of science and clinical practice as an explicit value. Shortly after, something called the *scientist-practitioner model* was born in 1949, which became the dominant model of training and practice for clinical psychologists. It meant that if you wanted to be the best possible clinical psychologist, then you needed to know how to be both a scientist and a clinician. Ideally, you would know how to integrate the two, so that the scientific literature could inform how you practice, and your clinical work could generate ideas for research. A clinician who knows how to read scientific literature is better able to avoid practicing pseudoscientific treatments that could be useless or harmful to patients. But there's more to being effective.

Clinicians also need to learn how to *be* with patients while guided by science. This is called *evidence-based practice*. It owes its history to a movement called *evidence-based medicine* (EBM), which became fully articulated in 1992. Its goal was to teach the idea that all health care professionals must engage in a delicate dance between three pillars: (a) the best available scientific evidence, (b) their own clinical experience and judgment, and (c) the values and preferences that patients hold. The essence of EBM acknowledges that scientific knowledge is limited and evolving but that science remains essential to guiding patient care. And as we learned in Chapter 4, it remains unethical to practice pseudoscience even if patients consent to its use.

Nowadays, all legitimate health care disciplines are philosophically based on evidence-based practice. Lifelong learning is a necessary, built-in duty because science is constantly advancing. For mental health professionals, this means that they need to keep apprised of scientific developments in the field and know how to deliver evidence-based treatments.

So, you might ask, what exactly is an evidence-based treatment? The short answer is that it's a type of psychotherapy or medication with scientific evidence to support its use. The real answer is that it's complicated.

The strongest way that scientists can tell if psychotherapies work is to use the same methods they'd use to test whether medications work: randomized controlled trials (RCTs). Treatments that perform well in RCTs earn themselves scientific points. The more times that treatment benefits are replicated in RCTs conducted by different research teams (to avoid conflicts of interest), the more confidence we gain in the treatment. Clinicians can look to professional organizations—such as the American Psychological Association, the American Psychiatric Association, or the UK National Institute for Health and Care Excellence—to help them evaluate the strength of evidence.

A heartbreaking certainty is that evidence-based treatments that look promising in the lab don't always help patients in the real world. There are plenty of reasons why. Sometimes clinicians and patients aren't a suitable match, and sometimes clinicians are unskilled. As discussed in Chapter 3, we also lack a complete understanding of mental illness and therefore how to best soothe and remove its symptoms. The very science of how we evaluate evidence-based treatments can also fall short. Here's how:

Imagine you're someone who suffers with depression. You respond to an ad requesting your participation in an RCT. You agree to volunteer because it will allow you to get treatment. The researchers tell you that the RCT will compare three groups of patients over 12 weeks. The first group will receive cognitive-behavioral therapy (CBT) for 12 sessions; the second group will receive thought field therapy (TFT) for 12 sessions (*one of the pseudoscientific treatments discussed in Chapter 7*); and the third group will be assigned to a waitlist control, which means they won't receive any treatment until after the 12 weeks are complete so that researchers can compare how people feel after CBT and TFT to a control group who remains depressed.

You've been assigned to the CBT group. Before your treatment starts, you fill out a bunch of questionnaires that assess your depressive symptoms. Then you do it twice more: after your treatment and 1 year later. Each time you fill out the questionnaires, you don't feel like much has changed. You notice you're a little less depressed, but you don't feel well enough to return to work or seek out a romantic relationship.

The researchers eventually contact you to tell you the results of the RCT. You're surprised to hear that both the CBT and TFT groups worked compared to the waitlist control. In other words, patients assigned to CBT and TFT reported feeling less depressed on average compared to the group of people who remained depressed and had to wait to get treatment. There were also no differences between the CBT and TFT groups in depression scores. How could any of this be?

For lack of a better word, figuring out whether treatments work is hard. RCTs come in many shapes and sizes, and they're one of the best ways to measure treatment effectiveness. But they also have limitations.

Arguably the biggest letdown with RCTs is that they deal in averages. In our hypothetical scenario, your depression didn't improve much after receiving CBT, while other people in your group improved much more than you. RCTs are fantastic at telling me which treatments work for the average patient among hundreds of thousands, but they're less helpful at telling me which treatment will be most effective for the individual patient sitting in my office.

Another common complaint against RCTs involves the questionnaires you filled out. They don't tend to be thorough or check in on how you're doing beyond 1 year, so it's hard to tell how long the benefit of a treatment lasts. More troublesome is that when ascertaining whether a treatment works, they often assess only for depressive symptoms, as opposed to other factors that really matter to patients, such as your readiness to return to work, how you function in social situations, or your overall quality of life. Mind you, these complaints aren't inherent flaws of how RCTs are designed, and they could be remedied by researchers by incorporating longer follow-up periods and more useful assessments.

There's a final double-edged sword of RCTs you should know about: Let's call it the *garbage in, garbage out* effect. In our hypothetical scenario, TFT performed just as well as CBT. But TFT is an undeniable pseudoscientific treatment because it operates from the assumption that mental illness can be treated by correcting imbalances in nonexistent human energy fields, whereas CBT is a well-established evidence-based treatment. As discussed in Chapter 7, TFT also makes use of CBT ideas and capitalizes on factors common to all talk therapies (which we'll learn about later). This means that the results of our RCT didn't consider TFT's lack of scientific plausibility. The benefits reported from

TFT have nothing to do with human energy fields—rather, they're misleading and show us the challenges of doing clinical research.

When scientists look only at the final outcomes of RCTs, they risk legitimizing pseudoscientific treatments. For this reason, many in the skeptic community have called for a greater focus on *science-based medicine* instead of *evidence-based medicine*. Science-based medicine *is* evidence-based medicine, but with an added alert begging us to pay attention to the idea of scientific plausibility, which we used in Chapter 7 to help us sort out unambiguous cases of pseudoscience from ambiguous ones.

Ignoring scientific plausibility makes it easier for the term "evidence-based" to be hijacked and promoted in the service of pseudoscience. Remember the pseudoscientific journals we learned about in Chapter 5, such as the *Journal of Evidence-Based Complementary & Alternative Medicine* and the *Journal of Evidence-Based Integrative Medicine*? The studies published in those journals are not doing patients any favors, to put it mildly, because they enable grifters to claim the mantle of science while only appearing to apply any sort of scientific rigor.

At the end of the day, RCTs are still the best way to tease out whether a treatment *causes* a beneficial or harmful effect, and no other research design is better for keeping our personal biases in check. They aren't panaceas and their results don't come with guarantees, but they remain one of our most powerful scientific tools to inform evidence-based practice.

Alphabet Soup for Your Mind

Aaron T. Beck died on November 1, 2021, 34 days after responding to my email. I had written in hopes of involving him in a book that I was coediting about mental health misinformation and pseudoscience. He responded by saying:

> Dear Jonathan,
>
> Thank you so much for your note. Your book sounds fascinating. Unfortunately, at the age of 100, I have limited amounts of energy so I will not be able to help.
>
> Best of luck,
> ATB

In hindsight, I feel foolish having bothered him. I knew he was 100 years old. In my defense, I was also starstruck. Beck was a psychiatrist who trained intensely in Freudian psychoanalysis during the middle of the 20th century. It was around that time that both clinical psychology and psychiatry began taking science more seriously. Beck wanted Freudian psychoanalysis to be accepted by the scientific community, so he started running some experiments to test out aspects of its theory.

For example, according to Freudian psychoanalysis, depression is caused by *inverted hostility*. This is the idea that a depressed person feels hostile or angry toward someone they care about, but they stuff those feelings down or repress them unconsciously because part of their mind deems them unacceptable. Once repressed, the hostility and anger invert and instead show up as depressed mood, suicidal wishes, self-criticism, and a negative outlook. Beck tested the idea by comparing the dreams of depressed and nondepressed people. If dreams were the "royal road to the unconscious," as claimed by Freud, then the dreams of depressed people should contain features of hostility. In Beck's experiment, it turned out that the dreams of people who were depressed actually contained less hostility than those of their nondepressed counterparts.

Several similar experiments later, Beck found himself increasingly disillusioned with psychoanalysis. In 1960, he was fed up. He didn't like how his tests kept failing and how psychoanalysis required patients to lie down on a couch during therapy. When instead he asked patients to sit up and have a conversation, he set himself on a course that would truly revolutionize mental health care. He became the father of CBT, one of the most scientifically supported approaches we have to address many different kinds of mental health concerns.

CBT sometimes gets a bad rap. That's bound to happen when you're among the most popular and scientifically investigated mental health treatments in the world. Its bruised reputation originates from at least two sources.

First, I've seen it recklessly pitched by clinicians as a panacea for all mental health concerns. This grinds my gears because, as we learned in Chapter 5, marketing anything as a panacea is a pseudoscientific red flag—and CBT is not even close to being a pseudoscience. This reckless handling of a valuable therapy does raise an important issue: Evidence-based treatments aren't cure-alls. They work better for some people and some mental health concerns and may be useless or harmful for others.

For example, a recent meta-analysis of 409 RCTs with 52,702 patients provided further high-quality evidence that CBT works for depression. Variants of CBT can also be spectacularly effective for anxiety disorders, addiction-related disorders, obsessive-compulsive disorder (OCD), and posttraumatic stress disorder (PTSD). Unfortunately, the evidence is weaker and more controversial with other kinds of mental health concerns, such as psychotic disorders and anorexia nervosa.

The other reason CBT is occasionally and unfairly condemned is due to confusion about what it entails. I've lost track of the number of times that patients have told me they've received CBT and then describe an experience that bore little resemblance to real CBT. This may sound harsh, but the reality is that some poorly trained clinicians falsely believe that reading straight out of a CBT treatment manual for six to 12 sessions constitutes good therapy. Clinicians aren't supposed to be robots who rigidly follow a script.

When working with a mental health professional, real CBT should feel like a smooth conversation. To help my students understand this point, I call it doing *ninja CBT*. It involves an engrossment in the principles of CBT to such an extent that it's no longer explicit—it's just a therapeutic language that patients and clinicians use together to facilitate psychological change.

More confusion about what CBT *is* can arise because CBT isn't just one thing. It has several advanced spinoffs that are adapted for addressing specific mental health concerns, such as *behavioral activation* for depression, *exposure and response prevention (ERP)* for OCD, and *prolonged exposure* and *cognitive processing therapy* for PTSD. There are also distinctly separate evidence-based therapies that grew out of CBT with slight shifts in theoretical underpinnings, such as *dialectical behavior therapy (DBT)* and *acceptance and commitment therapy*. It's beyond the scope of this book to detail these approaches in depth, but they do all share common core principles.

At the center of CBT is the idea that we can better understand our everyday life experiences by breaking them down into three interacting parts: thoughts, emotions, and behaviors. That means that what we think, how we feel, and what we do are all connected. In CBT, we use strategies to challenge how we think and change what we do to improve mental health and illness.

I often tell my patients that when we're engaging in CBT, we (perhaps fittingly) adopt the attitude of a scientist. We don't just accept our thoughts as facts, but rather we treat them as hypotheses to be explored, tested, and challenged. As discussed in Chapter 6, our minds are already biased toward thinking errors and deep-seated beliefs—this can be exacerbated during periods of intense distress and when we're experiencing mental disorders. So together, we gently strive to practice cultivating a more realistic, balanced, and helpful outlook. A common misconception about CBT is that it's all about positive thinking, rainbows and unicorns, and rose-tinted glasses. That's incorrect. In CBT, we're trying to increase our awareness of the unhelpfully biased lenses we're already wearing so that we can more easily take them off.

When Beck was developing CBT, he noticed the two styles of thinking we discussed in Chapter 6: the intuitive and analytical styles upon which Daniel Kahneman built his work. Recall that intuitive thinking feels impulsive and automatic, and it gets us into trouble. It makes us more susceptible to misinformation. We need to override it with analytical thinking that is more deliberate and reflective. In the same vein, intuitive thinking can lead to misinformation about our own experiences. Beck called it our *automatic thoughts*. In CBT, we challenge automatic thoughts and beliefs to gain a more complete view of reality. This connection between CBT and the broader scientific literature is just one way this form of therapy is granted scientific plausibility. To give you an introductory feel of the CBT approach, I'd like to show you the process behind one useful tool that I sometimes use with my patients called a *Thought Record*. You can read about it under the heading "How to Produce a Thought Record" on pages 213–216 in "Mind the Takeaways."

Beck justifiably moved on from Freudian psychoanalysis, which many authors have regarded as a classic pseudoscience. As we learned in Chapter 3, Freud developed his ideas at the turn of the 20th century and they blossomed in the American psychiatric community for decades. These days, Freudian psychoanalysis can still be found among some clinicians and mostly in university textbooks. If you've ever taken an introductory psychology class, you might remember concepts like the id, the ego, the superego, penis envy, and the Oedipus complex. I won't review these terms (but they're fun to Google) because they're old and outdated. But they're still taught, and in a rather unhelpful way, because they caricaturize and taint the image of Freudian psychoanalysis's modern offspring with a revamped name: *psychodynamic therapy*.

If CBT has an image problem, then psychodynamic therapy is in danger of being cancelled. Beck drifted away from Freudian psychoanalysis, but it gradually evolved without him into something useful. Modern-day psychodynamic therapists aren't mini-Freuds who are practicing a debunked pseudoscience. They sit on a mound of high-quality scientific evidence that is far removed from the more outlandish Freudian viewpoints. Some people in our Freud-averse world are surprised to learn that modern psychodynamic therapy is an evidence-based treatment. It just rarely gets airtime.

Jonathan Shedler is a psychologist who has taken academic and social media routes to correct these misunderstandings. In part, he blames the psychoanalytic community itself—that is, those devoted to practicing psychodynamic therapy—for decades of indifference to scientific research, a failing that continues to haunt the therapy's status. "Historically, psychoanalytic communities have been insular and inward facing. People who might otherwise be receptive to psychoanalytic approaches encounter impenetrable jargon and confusing infighting between rival theoretical schools," he writes.

While psychodynamic therapy is notorious for its use of confusing language, Shedler has a gift for making its concepts accessible. For example, he describes how esoteric-sounding terms like *object relations* and *attachment* just mean a focus on your relationship patterns and how you experience them. The term *transference* is fancy language for when a patient unwittingly views a clinician through the lenses of their early important relationships—for example, a person prone to distrusting others may view a clinician with suspicion.

The central tenets of psychodynamic therapy acknowledge the complexity of our minds: that much of mental life occurs outside of awareness; that we're often conflicted in our feelings, desires, and motivations; that our early life experiences influence who we are and how we perceive ourselves and the world; that we sometimes have a tendency to consciously and unconsciously avoid difficult experiences; and, just as we recognize in CBT, that our thoughts, emotions, and behaviors are connected in ways that give rise to mental health concerns. In psychodynamic therapy, clinicians work hard with patients to increase awareness of their deeply ingrained patterns of thinking and behaving, especially as those patterns play out in the therapeutic relationship itself.

If psychodynamic therapy sounds similar to CBT, that's because it is in many ways. Just as Kahneman's intuitive and analytical thinking styles are consistent with CBT theory and lend credence to its scientific plausibility, these styles can also be cast in the light of psychodynamic theory using its own language of *unconscious and conscious mental processes*. Both CBT and psychodynamic therapy also share commonalities with other evidence-based treatments, which we'll get to in the next section.

When patients arrive at my clinic, they typically don't care which treatment they receive. They just want to feel better because they're distressed and their functioning is extremely impaired—which, incidentally, are prerequisites before anyone can be diagnosed with a mental disorder as defined in the *Diagnostic and Statistical Manual of Mental Disorders*. In short, they're looking for psychological change. It's the job of clinicians to select the treatments they think will be most helpful. I've included a flavor of the most popular scientific approaches they should be drawing from in their practice under the heading "A Flavor of Evidence-Based Treatments" on pages 216–218 in "Mind the Takeaways." This list is in no way exhaustive because this book can't possibly cover the numerous psychotherapies and medications that are scientifically supported across different age groups, different formats (e.g., individual vs. group therapy), and different mental health concerns.

A Fly on the Wall in Therapy

When students shadow my psychotherapy sessions, they notice how rarely I give advice. Patients will ask questions like, "Should I leave my partner? Should I quit my job? Should I move across the country?" I empathize with the aching uncertainty of major life decision-making, but I can't answer those questions. I don't have the fortune-telling power to foresee what's in their best interests, nor would I want to abuse the power to remove their agency. That's not my job. Therapy isn't advice giving. It's coexploration leading to psychological change. And I discuss this with my patients in a way that clarifies roles, deepens our therapeutic relationship, and respects and supports their autonomy.

"I feel so relieved that you can be a flexible human in session," my students regularly tell me when learning how to do therapy. "Yes! That's the point," I tease. All too often students will put down their textbooks and arrive at my clinic with the misunderstanding that evidence-based practice is a stiff and machine-like process. That view shatters quickly when they need to throw out their session plan because a patient arrives in uncontrollable tears, intoxicated, or needing to go to the emergency department because they're expressing suicidal thoughts and plans.

Students eventually learn that real evidence-based practice is a process tailored to the needs of the patient, therapy goals are constantly revised, and patients themselves often take the lead. Therapy is a dance and is not merely providing psychoeducation or lecturing about treatments. Those treatments need to be delivered through the medium of human connection.

Once students discover that doing therapy is much thornier and more malleable than initially thought, they tell me they can finally breathe—which might seem paradoxical. But it's a rookie mistake to think that clinical expertise means knowing how to solve everyone's problems. Feeling unburdened by the pressure of having to know everything can free and inspire students to meld the discoveries of science with the art of healing.

In Lewis Carroll's 1865 book *Alice in Wonderland*, there's a scene where several characters become wet and need to dry themselves. As a solution, the Dodo bird calls for a race around the lake. After running for about half an hour until dry, the Dodo announces that the race is over. When the characters ask who won, the Dodo declares, "Everybody has won, and all must have prizes." This story came to represent an ongoing debate in psychotherapy research that has spanned nearly a century. Dubbed the *Dodo bird verdict*, it alludes to the idea that all psychotherapies are winners, as some scholars say that all are essentially the same in their effectiveness.

There are clear instances where the *Dodo bird verdict* is wrong. For example, studies show that some psychotherapies simply outperform others depending on specific mental health concerns. ERP for OCD is one such therapy that hands down outperforms others. We also know that scientifically plausible, evidence-based treatments work better than unambiguous and potentially harmful pseudoscientific treatments like past life regression therapy or conversion therapy.

But the *Dodo bird verdict* also gets something right. And it's crucial: Some psychotherapies share common factors that make them helpful. Marvin Goldfried is a distinguished psychologist at Stony Brook University who has been beating this drum for over half a century. "For well over 100 years, several hundred different schools of thought have been introduced into the field, each with a different theory and language system," he told me. "It's time for the field of psychotherapy to come of age. One way in which this can happen is the uncovering of common principles of change that exist in all approaches to treatment."

We already know what those common principles are.

Let's say that you experience severe social anxiety. If you go see a psychologist who practices psychodynamic therapy, they may tell you something like, "When you're afraid but then experience a situation you once feared without any harm, you won't immediately trust the outcome of your new experience.

But the second time, you will have a little less fear, and the third time still less, and so on."

If instead you see a psychologist who practices CBT and who unnecessarily uses heavy jargon, you might hear, "Let's extinguish the avoidance behavior by repeated exposure to the threatening stimuli under conditions to ensure the avoidance responses and the anticipated negative consequences don't occur."

Both psychologists are saying the same thing. Their techniques might be different, but they're both alluding to the idea that your social anxiety can be best treated by safely confronting anxiety-provoking situations. More broadly, this is one common principle that cuts across evidence-based treatments. Goldfried called it *encouraging corrective experiences.* Psychodynamic therapists call it that too, but they mostly encourage it within the confines of the therapeutic relationship. CBT therapists call it *exposure.* In everyday language, it just means encouraging new, more effective ways of behaving.

When my students feel overwhelmed with the vast array of evidence-based treatments to choose from, and when they're confused about where to go next in therapy to best help their patients, I always tell them: "Cultivate your human connection and lean on your evidence-based principles. That's the foundation of good therapy." These are the common helpful ingredients that can be found across all talk therapies:

- Having a strong relationship with a therapist
- Fostering motivation, hope, and positive expectations
- Increasing a person's awareness and insight
- Encouraging new, more effective ways of behaving
- Emphasizing constant reflection on those new, more effective ways of behaving
- Expressing empathy, nonjudgmental acceptance, and genuineness
- Where possible, having agreement on therapy goals

Above and beyond the specific techniques used in evidence-based treatments, research shows that these cross-cutting evidence-based principles contribute hugely to psychological change. Among the most powerful is building the therapeutic relationship. And it's a relationship like no other: It's not a friendship, it's not a mentorship, and it's obviously not an intimate or sexual relationship (though, reprehensibly, ethical boundary violations do occur). It's a unique relationship felt as an emotional bond, composed of privilege, trust, and unobscured safety, where a patient should be able to freely express absolutely anything and everything. Clinicians build and destroy these relationships based on how they converse with you. They succeed when they show you empathy, care, and belief in you as a person, rooting for you even as they attempt to address and repair any ruptures to the relationship that might unfold during psychotherapy; they fail when they're too rigid, confrontational, blaming, sarcastic, critical, or hostile. Without a strong therapeutic relationship, the other evidence-based principles vanish.

But some of these very principles can also explain why some people turn to alternative medicine and why pseudoscientific treatments can appear to work. Imagine if, instead of going to a psychologist to help with your social anxiety, you book an appointment with a "holistic mental wellness coach" who practices acupuncture. When you arrive, you're greeted by a personable smile and your senses are stimulated by apple pie–scented candles and the warmth of a cozy environment. You tearfully share your mental health journey, feeling seen and heard without judgment. You then receive acupuncture treatment and feel slightly better afterward. What happened?

You entered a placebo theater. Embraced with an ambience of positivity and the expectation of improvement, you improved. While the treatment you received had nothing to do with "meridians" or "balancing the energy of your life force," your "holistic mental wellness coach" took the time to get to know your story. They empathized with you, validated your concerns, and gave you much-needed hope.

But they didn't conduct a comprehensive psychological assessment to understand what was contributing to your mental health concerns because they weren't trained to know how. They won't be able to provide CBT-based exposure therapy, which is one treatment that maximizes your chances of experiencing relief from social anxiety down the road. You enjoy talking to them, but they were never trained to attend to ruptures in the therapeutic relationship should they arise, nor how to repair those ruptures. They might ask questions that seem relevant, but those questions aren't grounded in any theory and aren't directed with the psychotherapeutic precision needed to help increase insight into your mental health concerns. The crux: They've only accidentally stumbled upon enough evidence-based principles to lead you to some benefits, albeit haphazardly.

Good therapy requires the training and skills to deliver treatments that work in combination with knowing how to harness the helpful ingredients common to all talk therapies. When patients seek out alternative medicine practitioners who lack this training, they risk leaving their mental health in the hands of unreliable placebo effects, potentially harmful pseudoscientific treatments, and amateur management of the intimacy of therapy.

Thriving Afloat

It's the 20th psychotherapy session with me and you're still not feeling up to par. "Doc, my life is shit. Still no job. My kids hate me. I'm still drinking. And I feel heavy every morning. I can barely get out of bed," you confide. You've been battling an alcohol use disorder concurrent with a depressive disorder for almost 3 years now. I'm the third psychologist you've seen during that time. "What do I do?"

Unfortunately, this scenario is one I frequently wrestle with alongside my patients. The real world of mental health care saves lives, but it also consists of long and winding bumpy roads. You could participate in hundreds of hours of CBT or psychodynamic therapy, have a safe and secure therapeutic relationship with your mental health professional, and still end up feeling deflated by your perceived progress. In times like these, we troubleshoot and revert to basics.

A *stepped-care model* of mental health treatment is the idea that mental health can be improved by matching it with the intensity of treatment needed. In other words, if you're only experiencing mildly distressing mental health concerns but are still able to function and meet your responsibilities, you may only need to get your hands on some self-help materials like books, apps, or online programs to feel better. If instead you're experiencing severe psychopathology that feels overbearing and is interfering with aspects of your life, you may need a step-up in the intensity and focus of treatment, such as spending several nights in an inpatient psychiatric unit or attending a residential addiction program for weeks or months. While there's some debate in the research literature about the strength of the evidence behind organizing mental health care systems around formalized stepped-care models, the reality is that, loosely defined, they just make logical sense at the level of an individual patient: That is, the more you're suffering, the more intensive treatment you likely need, and vice versa.

My clinic happens to be designed for people who've already had treatment in the past and still aren't finding relief from their severe symptoms related to addiction and mental illness. Patients come to us when they need a step-up from their current treatment or their levels of mental distress and functioning have taken a hit after a period of recovery. Occasionally, however, a patient will come to us with no treatment history and no severe psychopathology. They need help with their mental health, not with mental illness.

Recall from Chapter 2 that mental health and illness aren't the same thing. Whereas mental illness refers to psychopathology, mental health is about thriving despite mental illness and the life stressors sapping our souls. It's getting back to a place of living with satisfaction, meaning, and self-care, even when we've already made lemonade with life's lemons and it still tastes rancid.

Easier said than done, I know. But it's worth appreciating that there are some things we can do on our own that generally benefit our mental health. This is one of the key components to mental health literacy: understanding how to obtain and maintain positive mental health. What are they?

I like to use the term *self-care* to describe these basics. Further, I break it down into two broad categories: biological and psychosocial. Biological self-care consists of the strategies we need to do on a regular basis to take care of ourselves physically, things like exercise; taking prescribed medications; going to dentists, eye doctors, and family physician appointments; eating nutritiously; getting restful sleep; etc. I used to run a weekly therapy group with a psychologist named Vanessa LaPrairie who referred to biological self-care as "taking care of our meat-suits." Some patients laughed, and some cringed, but they all got the idea.

In contrast, psychosocial self-care encapsulates the psychological and social ways we care for ourselves. It's practicing emotion regulation skills, enjoying hobbies and leisure activities, reciprocating in personal relationships, and connecting with community. Granted, the mind and body are intricately connected and so these two categories of self-care are artificial and overlapping, but they're useful because they point to different ways to improve our mental health.

As food for thought, I sometimes explore this question with my patients: "Which category of self-care do you think is more important, the biological or the psychosocial?" It's a question with multiple truths and no right answer. Both aspects of self-care play off each other. When you're feeling well mentally and connected to your community, you're more likely to want to exercise. At the same time, if you haven't exercised in a month, haven't slept well in weeks, and haven't eaten well either, you're less likely to want to socialize.

The message is that when life feels overwhelming and you don't know where to start, just pick any aspect of self-care. It doesn't matter which one. Both categories are pathways to recovery and regaining control.

The science is a fan of self-care. Research shows that social connection can reduce feelings of loneliness, which is a risk factor for physical and mental health problems. Poor-quality sleep is linked to several mental disorders, and finding ways to get restful sleep can improve symptoms. Exercise can be helpful in both preventing and treating common mental disorders, such as depressive and anxiety disorders. And the field of "nutritional psychiatry" is an emerging area of research showing that healthy diets (e.g., higher intake of fruits, vegetables, nuts, whole grains, legumes, and quality protein sources) can be helpful too.

As with the RCTs we learned about earlier, the scientific literature imparts a lesson in averages with self-care. No one is perfect: Everyone practices self-care at times, and everyone practices self-neglect. We just want to find a way to practice self-care *more* than we practice self-neglect. The science isn't a *prescription* telling us what we should be doing. It's not about guilting or shaming us if we fall short. It's merely a *description* of the evidence behind the options we can take to advantage ourselves.

Self-care lays a foundation for mental health, but it's not a silver bullet. I have plenty of patients who exercise daily with active social lives—and they still struggle. For those who experience eating disorders, overexercising can contribute to a worsening of symptoms that perpetuates body image concerns and interferes with their relationships. For some people who are depressed, self-care can feel like a daunting and unachievable feat of energy. Mental health can never be reduced to a one-size-fits-all approach.

Self-care can also be exploited by grifters. As we saw in Chapter 4, the wellness industry has been moralizing and selling exercise, sleep, and fad diet changes as a cure-all since the days of John Kellogg and Bernarr Macfadden. The commercialization of self-care means we need to be skeptical when perusing the self-help sections of our local bookstores and prudent when paying for mental health apps on our mobile Apple Stores. Although self-help apps can be useful tools that incorporate evidence-based treatment ideas, research shows that many are untested and lacking in quality. Worse, all forms of self-help materials can act as channels to promote pseudoscience.

At the other end of the stepped-care model spectrum, you or your loved one may be struggling with severe psychopathology and feel stagnant. Keep going. Keep addressing it with your mental health professional. Maybe there's more you can work on together, or maybe you need to end therapy and start anew, or maybe you need a medication review or extra resources such as peer support groups or a more intensive treatment program. This troubleshooting is the norm. Maintaining optimal mental health and recovering from mental illness are fluid expeditions. They aren't races with a finish line.

"Doc, I made it. I haven't used crack in three years. I don't bottle-pick anymore. I live in an apartment with my girlfriend. Life is good. I'll never forget when you visited me in the emergency department at my rock bottom, sitting at the foot of my bed as I cried." When patients keep going, these are the kinds of stories that I hear—and that keeps me going.

* * *

Consider the nirvana fallacy. It's the error in comparing realistic solutions to idealized perfect ones and then arguing that the realistic solutions should be dismissed because they're imperfect. It's important to avoid lobbing this fallacy at evidence-based mental health care. Yes, its solutions are drawn from incomplete science. We don't completely understand mental illness or why some people have an easier time recovering than others. We don't have perfect methods to even study what works and what doesn't. The solutions are necessarily tentative and fallible.

But the mental health professions know more than armchair psychologists like Andrew Tate. They're better than the alternatives presented in the wellness industry that are awash with pseudoscientific pipe dreams. There are medications and an alphabet soup of CBTs, ERPs, DBTs, and other approaches that have been shown to help for reasons that are scientifically plausible. Well-trained mental health professionals know how to distill and cultivate what works in therapy, and we know that self-care is paramount but no wonder drug.

Science doesn't care about marketing terms like *alternative medicine* or arbitrary distinctions between what is and what isn't considered *evidence-based*. I care about science, though—as do the mental health professions, because it's their saving grace. Their reliance on science is what allows them to learn and mature so that more people can experience mental health, as well as freedom from mental illness. Unfortunately, not everyone has access to real help or knows where to look. This book has been about using science to both protect ourselves and find hope. Let's pull it all together now.

9

Reclaim Your Mind

When Tamara was a child, she was repeatedly molested by a male neighbor. She didn't get to finish high school because she left home at age 12 to be sexually trafficked until she was 23 years old. At 14, she gave birth to a beautiful baby boy who was raised by her mother—he ignites a weighty but joyful fire in her eye whenever she talks about the kind of man he's become. At 15, her pimp introduced her to the crack cocaine that she would furiously inject and smoke consistently for years. At 40, she arrived in my clinic.

Tamara is one of the most intelligent, insightful patients I've ever had. If I'm honest, I remember frequently leaving our sessions feeling stunned. She had a gift for poetically articulating her pain while meaningfully connecting the dots of her traumatic experiences. It was awe-inspiring to join in her self-discoveries. We had a deeply strong therapeutic relationship for 3 years. She was winning the war against addiction and posttraumatic stress disorder (PTSD).

That's why when she messaged me years later to say that she got "caught up in some alternative medicine healing crap" and it took "a year to untwist" herself, I felt heartbroken. Had I failed her? Had the system failed her? How did she untwist herself?

"After we ended our therapy together, I still had other stuff. I didn't know where to go with my stuff. My soul was hungry for something spiritually. So, I just started Googling things and then found Amber," she told me. Tamara hadn't used crack for several years. She was super skilled at managing PTSD flare-ups, the symptoms of which had greatly diminished in intensity since our treatment together. Still, she was struggling. "I was saving up money to relapse. I figured I could either spend it on a bender or I could spend it on Amber's wellness retreat—I chose self-preservation because I knew addiction wasn't a solution."

I learned that Amber was running a wellness business, marketing herself with a few legally unprotected titles—an "evolutionary astrologer," "intuitive coach," and "holistic therapist"—and without any qualifications to offer mental health services. Her business sells individual healing sessions and group retreats. Her approach is theoretically manufactured with cobbled-together ideas from 12-step programs (see Chapter 7) and *evolutionary astrology*. I had to look that one up.

The astrologer Steven Forrest is one of its founders. In his book, *Yesterday's Sky: Astrology and Reincarnation*, he writes that evolutionary astrology is "A form of psychological astrology which is integrated with metaphysics. Where a twentieth century psychological astrologer might focus on the dynamics of childhood, the evolutionary astrologer focuses on the childhood of the soul—prior lifetimes, and the issues left unresolved from them." In other words, it's pseudoscience—and one endorsed by the actor Robert Downey Jr. on the front cover of Forrest's book.

As we talked, Tamara told me she paid $500 to attend Amber's 5-day retreat. After driving 10 hours to get there, she arrived at a lavish home situated on a lake. As other participants joined, Amber started smoking cannabis and encouraged others to do so as well. She explained that both cannabis and psilocybin were medicinal methods that were going to be used throughout their journey.

Tamara was open to this idea but had questions: "How does cannabis fit in therapeutically for intensive trauma and spiritual healing? How does microdosing psilocybin jibe with my psychiatric medications? What theories are you basing your approach on?" A talented clinician would jump at the opportunity to honestly engage Tamara in her questioning, using it as a moment to nurture their therapeutic relationship. In contrast, Amber was defensive and imposing. She retorted by saying that cannabis was her medicine and that she needed the freedom to use it herself to be an effective practitioner. She expressed scorn for psychiatric medications, opting instead for an "Eastern philosophical approach" to mental illness that embraces psychedelics. "Either get on board with what I'm fucking doing or get out," she said. Tamara decided to stay.

The next morning when participants woke up, they had breakfast and made light-hearted conversations. It was something Tamara felt she was missing and needed—a sense of community. Then Amber barged into their quarters like an "antagonistic tornado." As Tamara describes it, "She was very confrontational and violated my physical boundaries. She got right in my face. She said that if I'm not willing to heal, then I don't belong here. So, when I said I was leaving, she gaslit me. She said that I'd given up on myself and was quitting five minutes before the miracle happens."

The saying "Don't give up until the miracle happens" is an old trope that circulates in the 12-step community. Written in the Alcoholics Anonymous "Big Book," it means something like *keep going, and then things will get better*. Personally, I think the saying is wise. It's a nod to the notion that psychological growth is fed by persistence. Tamara disagreed in this case: "It's bullshit. You don't know when the breakthrough is happening." She has a point. The idea might help someone endure a long trek to healing, but it shouldn't be weaponized to keep a person from leaving an uncomfortable situation.

Nevertheless, Tamara stayed. Later that afternoon, Amber attempted something called a *psychodrama*. It's a kind of experiential psychotherapy that was developed by psychiatrist Jacob L. Moreno in 1921. In a group format, participants are supposed to re-enact their traumatic experiences or relationship problems by role-playing a scene. The clinician is the director, one participant is the main character known as a protagonist, and the other participants play the role of people or objects in the protagonist's life, or even as their thoughts, emotions, and behaviors. Psychodrama enjoyed its heyday in the 1950s, but you won't find that it's practiced much in mainstream mental health care nowadays. While it's not so far-fetched to be deemed scientifically implausible, it doesn't have the research support to back it up. There's a lack of studies that evaluate the effectiveness of psychodrama, and the small literature that exists takes the form of teachings that are composed of mostly anecdotal evidence, clinical vignettes, and case illustration reports.

Even if Amber was a trained and licensed mental health professional, the use of psychodrama would be ethically dubious given its lack of supporting evidence. It's flatly wrong to use it without any qualifications at a wellness retreat among people with varying types and severity of mental health concerns. And it's just reckless to use it immediately after instructing people to smoke cannabis, which is what Amber did. Tamara hadn't used cannabis in a long time because she found that it interfered with her recovery. But on day 1 of the retreat, she conceded to Amber's instructions and went along with the combined psychodrama plus cannabis treatment, telling me that it felt invasive and compounded her mental anguish.

"On day 2, I woke up with a panic attack. I was hyperventilating on the floor, feeling my heart palpitating, sobbing uncontrollably, and unable to regulate," Tamara told me. As a remedy, Amber gave her a glass of water containing a mushroom cap. When Tamara pushed back, Amber claimed that it was "just a microdose of psilocybin" and that it would help. Tamara reluctantly drank the water. "Two hours later, I was at war with myself."

Tamara understood that the psilocybin was supposed to help participants find their purpose in life. To that end, Amber also instructed participants to jump into the frigid lake to *sur-face*, meaning that they would *face* their purpose after jumping and swimming to the *sur*face of the water. To me, this sounded confusing at first; but it's less confusing if we recall from Chapter 5 that a classic propaganda tactic used in alternative medicine is to invent, distort, and mislead with language (e.g., *dis-ease*). As Tamara put it, "Amber often did this with language."

So, Tamara stood up, walked down a 100-foot pier, and jumped into the mountain lake water. She said she almost died. "It was traumatic and intense. I didn't surface with a purpose other than getting myself out of that freezing lake. I couldn't get up. It took all my physical strength, and everyone was just watching me, not helping. I finally flopped up on the dock like a dead fish." Tamara told me she felt foolish. When she was young, her mother would rhetorically ask whether she would jump off a bridge at the request of a stranger—and here she was, doing almost exactly that.

The participants were conforming to Amber's approach. She had them watch the movie *Fight Club* as a model of her kind of healing: "We don't talk about what happens here to the outside world," Amber warned. To Tamara, it felt "cult-y," because what participants said and did were tightly controlled.

For the remainder of the retreat, Tamara sat in silence. She felt beaten down, dismissed, and isolated. But she also allowed herself to surrender to the process and left the retreat feeling like she had a spiritual mission to accomplish. "Amber had groomed me. She knew that I always wanted to use my traumatic experiences to help people. So, she hit me in my soft spots—she convinced me that I too could become a healer and benefit the masses."

Tamara joined Amber on three more retreats costing her thousands of dollars. She was tasked with recruiting participants, including survivors of sexual exploitation. "Amber wanted my expertise for this population of wounded souls," Tamara told me. It wasn't until the fourth retreat that she finally understood she'd been taken for a ride. The wakeup call occurred when Amber once again became physically confrontational and suddenly left in the middle of the retreat, abandoning Tamara in a rural area with no ride home. "I felt like I was 16 again, calling my mom to pick me up after I had been abused by my pimp. It was dreadful," she told me.

I found Tamara's wellness-retreat story troubling not only because of my personal connection to her but also because it spoke to so many topics I've touched on in this book: her desperation for spiritual fulfillment that was temporarily quelled by the seduction of pseudoscience (Chapter 1); her use of science and mental health literacy skills to question Amber's approach (Chapter 2) and anti-psychiatry beliefs (Chapter 3) and qualifications (Chapter 4); Amber's language manipulation tactics (Chapter 5); the uncanny resemblance to Kirby Brown's tragedy, only Tamara escaped with her life (Chapter 6); and falling victim to pseudoscientific practices (Chapter 7), despite prior experience with evidence-based treatment (Chapter 8).

In true Tamara fashion, she didn't mince her words when recounting the gravity of her ordeal: "I question whether I should be alive given the convoluted fuckery that I experienced at the hands of alternative medicine." She told me she felt compassion for Amber, who disclosed her own mental health concerns during the retreat, but remained firm against the idea that lived experience alone is enough to offer mental health services. "Anyone can call themselves an alternative medicine practitioner and get some legitimacy. It's wrong. It's not a game. We aren't test subjects. I entrusted a practitioner with my darkness and ended up doing a disservice to myself. It worsened my mental health. There's no recourse for me now. No governing body to report to."

Tamara not only survived but also found a way to reclaim her mental health. When I asked how she untwisted herself, she described a few strategies. First, she noted that the exposure therapy we did together years ago was effective for treating her PTSD symptoms, and so she sought another psychologist with training in evidence-based practice to reinvigorate the exposure work, as well as to help her practice emotional coping skills derived from dialectical behavior therapy. "Fake help is so easily accessible. Google is important, but it must be done right," she said. "People need to research their practitioner, and if nothing exists on the person or they aren't a real licensed professional then that's not good."

Second, she worked tenaciously to figure out what compelled her to go against her "better judgment." "I did a lot of journalling, crying, and sifting fact from fiction in relation to my experiences, trying to understand why I kept falling for this crap. I realized there were subtleties, it felt covert and insidious, and the crazy didn't come all at once—it was slow. In hindsight, there were plenty of red flags on the field."

Lastly, she returned to self-care. She reconnected with her goals, values, community, and friendships. "I had friends continually remind me who I am. I'm not a sucker. I was a warrior before this and still am."

* * *

Tamara shouldn't have been put in a position to easily turn to alternative medicine in the first place. I find it hard not to blame myself. We initially agreed to end our therapy together due to Tamara's substantial progress in therapy combined with the systemic pressures on my clinic. That is, I work in the public sector, and as such, my hospital clinic—and all similar mental health clinics—are at the mercy of government allocation of resources. Practically, this means that it isn't feasible at our clinics to see all patients continuously beyond certain timelines, particularly once they experience benefits from treatment like Tamara did—and even when there's more work that could always be done. In fact, our work together for 3 years extended 2 years beyond the recommended timeline. While many patients don't need or want ongoing therapy beyond 1 year, many do, and they're not always best served the way our system is structured.

However, all things considered, the Alberta public mental health care system in which I practice is arguably one of the best in the world: We have free access to care with an army of skilled mental health professionals delivering evidence-based treatments around the clock. The same can't be said for other public systems worldwide, particularly in the United States, where the situation is far worse. For example, the U.S. Government Accountability Office has reported shortages of mental health care providers, meaning that potentially millions of Americans can't access care when they need it and are placed on long waitlists whether they have coverage for services through their public or private health plans. The broken U.S. mental health care system is even more dire for minority and underprivileged groups, as research shows they're less likely to both seek and receive services.

During the process of writing this book, I struggled with how to address these global systemic and cultural barriers to receiving evidence-based mental health care. Many people turn to alternative medicine because they can't access quality treatment. The truth is that I don't have any silver bullets to offer as solutions at the structural and systemic levels. I'm not a public health policy expert, nor am I a journalist, sociologist, political scientist, or economist. As such, it's beyond the scope of this book to deep dive into these problems, and I refuse to feign expertise.

But from the perspective of a full-time practicing clinical psychologist with a foot in academia who works at the level of the individual, the best thing I can offer is guidance on bulletproofing yourself against pseudoscientific grift and seeking out best-in-class mental health care that is within your control.

Taming Your Google Search Bar

I have what some might call a weird habit. At least once a week, I covertly voyage into the darkest bowels of the wellness industry. It involves joining alternative medicine social media groups, following the work of various wellness influencers, surfing alternative medicine clinic websites, and talking to members in the community. This habit allows me to better understand the viewpoints and marketing strategies of those who peddle pseudoscience.

When Tamara found Amber online, she regrettably recognized only in hindsight numerous warning signs. Those are encompassed in the pseudoscientific red flags and alternative medicine tropes and propaganda tactics that you learned about in Chapter 5. My advice is to cement them into your mind. Take a picture of the relevant pages in this book and post them on your fridge if you must. That might sound excessive, but it could very well save you immense pain and even your life—as well as your bank account.

When searching for quality mental health information online, it's just as crucial to recognize what to avoid as it is to know what to seek. The very first step is to decide what kind of material you're looking for—and it's okay if that's not immediately obvious. Here are some questions worth considering:

Am I looking for . . .

- Ways to improve mental health on my own?
- Information about the nature and treatment of mental disorders?
- The assistance of local mental health professionals?
    - A psychological assessment?
    - General counseling?
    - Psychotherapy for mental health concerns?
    - Psychiatric medications?

Once you obtain a firmer grasp on the kind of information needed, you can scour the internet more pointedly. If you're hunting for factual information about mental health and illness, then you want to ensure that your sources are credible. But how can you tell between a credible source and one that's shady?

One option is to go directly to primary sources. This means using your science and mental health literacy skills to read scientific journals. Some people will feel more comfortable and equipped in this endeavor than others, and unfortunately, not everyone has access to these sources, many of which exist in online databases behind paywalls.

One risk of delving into the research literature to get your information is that interpretation can be difficult, depending on the complexity of the topic and the sophistication of the studies. An additional risk is the potential for extracting misinformation from low-quality journals and the pseudoscientific ones that we learned about in Chapter 5. Engaging with the research literature isn't an easy process, especially during periods of heightened distress. For these reasons, you probably want to compare the information you discover from primary sources with the information communicated by professional associations.

Major psychological and psychiatric professional associations are generally reliable. These are associations composed of mental health professionals who are devoted to advocating for the science and evidence-based practice of their disciplines. Nationally, in Canada, this would be the Canadian Psychological Association and the Canadian Psychiatric Association; in the United States, it would be the American Psychological Association and the American Psychiatric Association. Canadian provinces and U.S. states also have their own associations, as do other countries and jurisdictions.

Professional association websites may contain some information that's too advanced for nonprofessionals, but they'll also include resources—such as position papers and fact sheets—in easy-to-read language for the public. If you can't find what you're looking for, then reach out. It might feel awkward, but proactively contacting your national or local associations with your questions could direct you to exactly what you need. No question about mental health or the nature and treatment of mental illness is off limits.

The last place you want to look for trustworthy information is in those bowels of the wellness industry—I'd prefer not to see you there during my weekly escapades. Avoid getting your information from threads in online forums and social media groups that flaunt alternative medicine buzzwords (e.g., *holistic, natural, toxins, detox*). Beware of the blogs of social media influencers, especially if they're selling merchandise or health products (e.g., supplements, fad diets). Be suspicious of celebrity wellness brands (e.g., Goop, Poosh). Run from clinic websites waving the flags of *integrative medicine, functional medicine, complementary and alternative medicine*, and *naturopathic medicine*. These are spaces where you're unlikely to find credible, unbiased information about mental health and illness.

You might instead want to find someone to help you or your loved ones with mental health concerns. The resources available will depend on where you live. A good first step is to book an appointment with your family physician, if you have one. Family physicians are like the Swiss Army knives of medicine—they're helpful in navigating a wide range of fields. Sharing your mental health concerns with them can initiate a referral to a mental health professional or a mental health clinic, depending on your needs.

A caveat: Some family physicians have more mental health training than others. I would caution against accepting psychiatric medications from them without a thorough psychological assessment. As discussed in Chapter 3, medication can be lifesaving, but overprescribing is also a real problem, and you don't want to be put on medication unnecessarily. As someone who works in a hospital clinic that specializes in concurrent addiction and mental disorders, I see this very serious error too often, as our team spends considerable time safely de-prescribing and tapering people off their medications, particularly those in the benzodiazepine class, which are most commonly prescribed for concerns related to anxiety and sleep (e.g., alprazolam, clonazepam, lorazepam, etc.), as well as the opioid class, which are most commonly prescribed for pain (e.g., codeine, hydrocodone, oxycodone, etc.). Self-advocacy is important: So, when in doubt, request a referral to a mental health professional.

You may also choose to self-refer to a mental health professional in private practice. Here's another point at which those professional association websites may come in handy. For example, the American Psychological Association offers a Psychologist Locator tool, and the Canadian Psychological Association provides links to provincial associations with their own search tools.

Beyond psychologists and psychiatrists, other kinds of mental health professionals can be invaluable in your treatment plan too. Certain types of social workers and nurses are trained to provide psychotherapy, and I personally know many who are incredibly skilled. All evidence-based mental health professionals share a philosophical allegiance to a biopsychosocial model of care, meaning they understand that mental health and illness have biological, psychological, and social aspects that need to be addressed. While some professions may focus more heavily on one aspect, a solid treatment plan involves attending to each as necessary and may need to involve a team of professionals.

Recall that when I spoke to Tamara, she warned about the negative consequences of poorly researching your potential practitioner. It's a sage warning. Even when you use the search tools from professional associations, you want to exercise due diligence by carefully examining the credentials of those you plan to trust with your mental health.

Some practitioners will have personal websites. Good ones will feature their educational background, professional license number, and the exact kinds of mental health services they offer. They'll describe their clinical experience and areas of expertise, also being careful to outline their areas of nonspecialization for which they can't assist. Scan these websites for pseudoscientific red flags and alternative medicine tropes. A telltale sign that you've wandered onto grift territory is if you see a monster list of unrelated conditions across all ages that the practitioner purports to treat, from childhood developmental disabilities to gastrointestinal problems, addiction, psychosis, memory problems, chronic pain, and palliative care. No one is that capable or specialized. All mental health care professionals have areas of competence and incompetence.

It goes without saying that you want your practitioner to be licensed. But you also want to be vigilant about phony credentials. Some non–mental health professionals will use meaningless, unprotected titles (e.g., *clinical psychotherapist*) and then dress them up by obtaining fake credentials or registering with pseudoscientific associations. For example, the "Spiritual Regression Therapy Association (SRTA)" has a website containing a Find a Certified Therapist tool. It links to practitioners trained by the "Past Life Regression Academy," which is accredited by the "International Board of Regression Therapy" and recognized by the "UK Complementary and Natural Healthcare Council." This professional posturing makes it sound like there's legitimate training and credentialing required to become a bona fide past life regression therapist. There isn't. And it cloaks the pseudoscientific practice of past life regression therapy in an air of reputability. It can be very easy to fall prey to such fake certifications that resemble the qualifications legally issued by regulated health professions.

Not all qualified practitioners will have a personal website or a professional digital footprint. If they don't, then it's worth contacting them directly to inquire about their credentials. You may want to dig deeper in a more personal way to find out exactly how they can meet your mental health needs.

Let the Buyer Be Questioning!

Even though Tamara deeply regretted caving into Amber's pseudoscientific approach to trauma and spiritual healing, she didn't acquiesce silently. She challenged Amber with her science and mental health literacy skills by asking the appropriate questions to vet Amber's competence, despite the fact that her queries weren't well received. When searching for a potential practitioner, it's important to remember that it's okay—in fact, it's encouraged—to be curious about their knowledge and methods. I often tell my patients that in therapy, they're the driver of their treatment plan and I'm the passenger who may act as a guide. But I'll fail to effectively navigate if I'm unfamiliar with the terrain.

I've mentioned that when people come to therapy, they often just want to feel better and don't care about the approach of the practitioner. Mental health professionals have an ethical obligation to practice evidence-based care. Unfortunately, we've learned how that ideal is far removed from the realities of everyday practice. The burden shouldn't fall on patients to shop for practitioners as if they were purchasing an appliance. But it does, and at the end of the day your mental health is on the line. You want to make sure your appliance works.

I empathize with the frustration of having to put in the work to find effective care when one is feeling at their lowest and most vulnerable. To make it easier, it can be helpful to have some questions in your back pocket and ready to go for an initial call with a potential practitioner or even your first couple of appointments. Here are some suggestions to carry with you:

- Can you please tell me about your credentials?
    - o Are you licensed by a regulatory body that issues a protected title, such as a psychologist, psychiatrist, social worker, or nurse?
    - o What kinds of mental health concerns do you specialize in treating?
    - o What kinds of mental health concerns are beyond your scope of practice?
- Can you please tell me about your clinical experience?
    - o How long have you been licensed and practicing?
    - o Lately, I've been feeling ______________ (e.g., *sad, depressed, lonely, anxious, irritable, angry, withdrawn*, etc.) and I've been experiencing problems with ____________ (*my friendships, romantic relationship, employment, alcohol, drugs, sleep, eating, isolating, getting out of bed,*

meeting my responsibilities, etc.). Have you had any experience in helping people with my concerns?

- Are you familiar with evidence-based practice?
  - o What does it mean to you?
  - o What kinds of evidence-based treatments do you use?
    - Can you please tell me a bit about the science behind them?
    - Do you practice from a particular theoretical orientation, such as cognitive-behavioral or psychodynamic?
  - o What can I expect our therapy together to look like?
    - Is there a certain number of sessions?
    - Do you provide individual and/or group therapy?
    - What are your fees and attendance policy?
- If necessary, how would you involve other health professionals in my treatment, such as family physicians, dietitians, other types of mental health professionals, and/or other specialists?
- What's your opinion on the role of psychiatric medications in a patient's care?

The point of these questions is to use them as a cheat sheet to get a feel for your potential practitioner. It's obviously not to interrogate them in a disrespectful or accusatory manner. Most skilled mental health professionals would welcome your inquiries and would embrace the opportunity to start building rapport and a therapeutic relationship with you.

Don't be afraid to get technical. For example, if you experience obsessive-compulsive disorder, ask them about their training in exposure and response prevention (see Chapter 8). Ask them their opinions about the benefits and harms of psychiatric medications or the ethics of practicing clear cases of pseudoscientific treatments. A practitioner who immediately vilifies psychiatric medications or reveals that they practice pseudoscience is not a practitioner I would trust with the mental health of my loved ones.

To a well-trained mental health professional, these questions are easy to answer and won't be considered insulting. They also give you a chance to gauge their ability to empathize, understand, validate, and listen to you. Recall from Chapter 8 that having a strong therapeutic relationship is one of the most important factors contributing to a helpful outcome. If you don't feel like it's a good match, then you're not obligated to seek their assistance. In a very real sense, you're hiring someone to do a vital job. You're allowed to interview elsewhere too, and you don't need to settle if your questions aren't answered to your satisfaction.

The Best Offense Is a Good Defense

"What on Earth is TikTok?" is a question I asked myself when the app first launched in 2018. I quickly discovered that it's a social media platform allowing users to create and share short videos to entertain, connect, and learn. When it first came out, it mostly featured amateur comedy interspersed with people singing and dancing. It now has over 1 billion monthly users worldwide and is firmly embedded in popular culture. Its content has evolved to become a repository of rich information on pretty much any topic. One such topic is mental health. If you have the TikTok app on your phone, you can search the hashtag #mentalhealth and see for yourself that it's been mind-blowingly accessed over 107 billion times.

Clicking on the hashtag will take you to videos with mental health–related content. But how useful and accurate are the videos? Marco Zenone is a public health researcher who studies misinformation and online portrayals of health and wellness issues. He wanted to answer those exact questions. When he asked whether I'd be interested in joining his team, I didn't hesitate.

We took a sample of the top 1,000 TikTok videos with the hashtag #mentalhealth from a specific timeframe in 2021 and then analyzed the content. Most videos involved users sharing their personal stories, thoughts, or perspectives, and over one-third contained advice or information presented as factual. When we analyzed the videos with advice and information—which were watched over 1 billion times—we found that 67% could be considered useful, but 33% were misleading. Some of the misleading videos parroted anti-psychiatry tropes, such as the idea that medications aren't helpful and "are for profit only." Alarmingly, the misleading videos also received more views, likes, comments, and shares than ones we classified as useful. Our findings—currently submitted for publication—are consistent with other studies showing that TikTok videos contain high amounts of misinformation about more specific health topics, such as attention-deficit hyperactivity disorder, diabetes, prostate cancer, and Covid-19.

TikTok is only one gargantuan source of mental health misinformation where online creators can—unintentionally or not—play expert and therapist to billions of users. We are at a point in human history where we have access to the best available information at our fingertips, and yet it doesn't lead to better-informed health decisions because that information is drowned out by a rival proliferation of emotionally charged fake science news, conspiracies, alternative facts, and social media echo chambers. How can people find quality mental health care while shielding themselves against such a bombardment of damaging noise? I hope I've given you some direction.

We learned in Chapter 6 that people fall for mental health misinformation and pseudoscientific grift for many complex and interacting reasons. For most of us, many of these reasons are beyond our control. Unless you have undue power over the way that social and popular media companies amplify misinformation or over the business practices in the wellness industry, it makes little sense to stress about how to tackle these influences head on. Instead, I've maintained throughout this book that, contrary to the old adage, the best offense is a good defense.

Pseudoscience and wellness aren't going anywhere. I find that fact deeply unsettling. But it's rejuvenating to know that we can affect their demand. A person who views their mental health with a scientific lens is advantaged. Grifters hold less power over those who can see through their charades.

Defending ourselves is like putting on layers of medieval body armor. Honed science and mental health literacy skills are the boots that keep us grounded in evidence. The body plates represent our vigilance to pseudoscientific warning signs and alternative medicine advertising. The helmet symbolizes introspection, which involves practicing intellectual humility and critically attending to our thinking errors, logical fallacies, socially influenced belief systems, and risky personality proclivities. We reclaim our mental health with a sword made from perseverance, couched in an understanding that evidence-based mental health care necessarily provides imperfect solutions rooted in an evolving science.

* * *

Tamara was able to reclaim her mental health in a feat of dogged determination. If you knew her spirit, you would expect nothing less. Her redemption story prevails in a sea of others. On social media, people take the liberty to share their ordeals with me all the time. I'm constantly reminded of the relief they experience once they've broken free from the lure of grift. I'm told, "I can't believe I fell for that nonsense and wasted all that money," or "I can't believe it took so long to get a real diagnosis and find a therapist that actually helps." Hearing these stories provides much-needed respite from the tragedies, such as "I'm angry that a close friend was sold snake oil and lost his life in a downward spiral of schizophrenia."

Knowing when, where, and how to get help is a core component of mental health literacy. And it's difficult. With a magic wand, we'd be able to increase access and availability of evidence-based mental health care to everyone. Mental illness stigma would be an afterthought. We'd fully understand the nature of psychopathology and our treatments would be much more helpful. We'd see the regulatory bodies of health professions step up and crack down on cases of clear-cut pseudoscientific practices.

Reality is more dismal, as access to quality care is limited and gaps exist in our knowledge. The wellness industry entices us but makes us sicker. It doesn't have to, though.

I wrote this book to empower people to take their mental health into their own hands. I wanted to teach the language of pseudoscientific grift so that you know when it's spoken. This is a kind of mental health support I'm unable to provide in the role of clinician.

People sometimes wonder how I respond to patients when they ask me about alternative medicine treatments. I explain that my approach to science communication is quite different from clinical work. It must be. Clinically, the therapeutic relationship matters the most.

For instance, if a patient requests past life regression therapy, I will empathically decline, explaining that I cannot ethically practice a potentially harmful pseudoscientific treatment that is beyond my scope of practice. I will validate their thoughts and beliefs, and we will explore them together. I will also respect their autonomy to seek that type of treatment elsewhere while continuing to offer the best therapy based on the best evidence to the best of my ability. As we've learned, that patient may even report benefits from past life regression therapy due to placebo effects and factors common to all talk therapies. For that patient, I'm thrilled.

For the many patients duped and harmed by pseudoscientific practices, I'm livid. Alternative medicine does more harm than good on average—on the grand scale beyond the individual patient. Sometimes, it's fatal. I've made that case in this book. Everyone, including grifters, generally deserves to be treated with kindness and respect—ideas don't, especially terrible ones. Tolerating pseudoscience in our culture is not a victimless crime. It's an intellectual crime with grave consequences. My hope is that by minding the science, you feel better prepared to safeguard and enrich your mental health.

Mind the Takeaways

Anti-Psychiatry Tropes and Corrections

Anti-Psychiatry Tropes	Corrections
Psychiatry still promotes the "chemical imbalance" hypothesis to explain mental illness.	The "chemical imbalance" explanation was an early and incorrect way to make sense of the effectiveness of medications that alter neurotransmitters in the brain. Currently, the biochemical mechanisms of mental illness and how treatments work are still being researched.
It isn't ethical to use a medication if one doesn't understand exactly how it works.	This has never been a principle in the medical world. The efficacy and safety of medications are very often established before mechanisms of action are fully understood and they guide future scientific work.
Psychiatric medications are harmful.	All medical interventions can cause harm, including surgery, medications, psychotherapy, and recommendations to exercise. Treatments must be understood and explained in terms of their risks and benefits relative to prognosis without treatment. This is the foundation of informed consent.
Psychiatric medications don't work.	There are a range of different psychiatric medications used to treat different conditions, each with varying levels of efficacy compared to placebo.
Psychiatric medications only mask symptoms and cause emotional numbing.	Medications are often used alongside psychotherapy to address the causes of mental health concerns from a biological, psychological, and social perspective. Scientific evidence shows that emotional numbing can occur as a side effect of medications but that it's different from effectiveness. For example, medications can improve depressive symptoms that cannot be regarded as merely "numbing," such as restoring lack of energy, lack of pleasure, loss of appetite, and insomnia.
Psychiatric diagnoses are made by a *Diagnostic and Statistical Manual of Mental Disorders* (DSM) checklist.	Sound diagnosis requires thorough investigation, interview, collateral history, objective examination, and sometimes "ruling out" medical disorders and other psychiatric issues. The DSM is not the "Bible" of psychiatry. It's one tool used in an assessment and an imperfect rough guide that continues to be revised.

Anti-Psychiatry Tropes	Corrections
Psychiatrists practice "biological psychiatry" and only care about pushing medications.	Modern psychiatry is a medical subspecialty that seeks to understand mental illness by integrating the biological, psychological, and social aspects of one's life. Psychiatry was actually ahead of most medical fields in understanding the impact of psychological and social factors on people's health. Well-trained psychiatrists practice conservative prescribing and de-prescribing when appropriate, constantly preaching "skills over pills."
Mental health professions seek to "medicalize" ordinary emotional distress.	The boundary between health and disease is "fuzzy" across all areas of medicine. Psychiatry focuses on emotional suffering and impairments to functioning, whether distress is an expected reaction to a situation or not. Well-trained psychiatrists remain vigilant about overdiagnosis and overprescribing.
Mental illness doesn't exist.	The definitions and boundaries of particular mental disorders fluctuate over time, reflecting our evolving understanding of their nature. Currently, mental disorders are best understood as clusters of symptoms that co-occur in patterns that can be reliably recognized to help guide evidence-based treatment approaches.
Psychiatrists ignore lifestyle changes, such as diet and exercise.	Sometimes lifestyle changes are insufficient on their own to address the complexity of mental illness. Nevertheless, well-trained psychiatrists regularly incorporate lifestyle interventions during treatment planning, often in conjunction with other health care professionals.

Nine Red Flags of Pseudoscience

Red Flag	What It Sounds Like
1. Explain away negative findings (i.e., overuse of ad hoc hypotheses)	"Your horoscope didn't work this time because you didn't think positively enough when you read it."
2. Absence of self-correction	"Sure—maybe Scientology hasn't changed much since L. Ron Hubbard's writings, but it still has undiscovered potential!"

Red Flag	What It Sounds Like
3. Evasion of peer review	"They don't publish their results in top-tier, peer-reviewed scientific journals because Western medicine has brainwashed us to believe that randomized controlled trials (RCTs) are the only kind of evidence."
4. Emphasis on confirmation rather than refutation	"I don't care if you think the Amazing James Randi has thoroughly debunked telekinetic spoon bending. Those people at the workshop swear it isn't a magic trick!"
5. Reversed burden of proof	"No! YOU prove to ME that isn't an alien-operated UFO."
6. Claims divorced from the broader scientific literature (i.e., absence of connectivity)	"Science doesn't have all the answers! It can't explain how past life regression therapy uses ideas about reincarnation to help treat posttraumatic stress disorder."
7. Elevation of anecdotal evidence	"I received energy healing and happen to feel better afterward; therefore, it works."
8. Use of science-y sounding language	"Once the diagnosis using quantum mechanics is completed, current treatments revert to biochemistry instead of using treatments involving the subtle energies that made the original diagnosis." (From an actual published article on energy medicine that is now retracted)
9. Absence of boundary conditions	"Why, of course detoxification diets can treat depression, anxiety, addiction, attention-deficit hyperactivity disorder, chronic pain, marital conflict, glaucoma, Covid-19, laziness, and heartburn—and it can do so in adults, children, infants, dogs, cats, and horses."

Alternative Medicine Tropes and Corrections

Alternative Medicine Tropes **"Unlike in mainstream mental health care, alternative medicine treatments . . ."**	**Corrections**
"Address the root cause"	People who promote alternative medicine often abuse the phrase "addressing the root cause" when they talk about treating mental health or illness. The problem is not so much that "addressing the root cause" is wrong—in fact, treating multiple causes is a mainstay of mainstream mental health care. We treat multiple causes of a person's mental health concerns all the time with both psychotherapy and medication. The problem is that in alternative medicine, a pseudoscientific or false "root cause" is often targeted. For example, you might see an advertisement that a person's posttraumatic stress disorder symptoms can be treated by addressing the trauma they experienced in a past life using past life regression therapy. Or you might read about using Reiki to treat the "root cause" of a person's depressive symptoms, which is mistakenly believed to be their unbalanced energy. The Medical Medium has alluded to heavy metals and Epstein-Barr viruses as the root causes of anxiety. The truth is that alternative medicine practitioners rarely possess the qualifications to evaluate the causes of mental health concerns, let alone diagnose or recommend treatment.
"Don't mask the symptoms"	Similar to the trope above, it's common to hear that "mainstream mental health care providers only want to cover up the symptoms, not prevent or treat the problem itself." This charge trivializes the complexity of mental health concerns and distills them down to an oversimplified state that can then be treated with a pseudoscientific approach. The insult inherent to these kinds of tropes is that mainstream mental health care providers are ignorant and only know how to treat symptoms.
"Are safer"	Just as all medical interventions can cause direct harm—including surgery, medications, psychotherapy, and recommendations to exercise—so too can treatments touted as alternative medicine. Pseudoscientific treatments can also indirectly cause harm by delaying effective treatment and lead to worsening symptoms. And that doesn't even cover their harm at the level of public health as fixtures in our culture in the largely unregulated wellness industry where many are not tested for safety.

Alternative Medicine Tropes **"Unlike in mainstream mental health care, alternative medicine treatments . . ."**	**Corrections**
"Use the placebo effect"	The placebo effect occurs when a person's symptoms improve following an inert or sham treatment. This trope sounds like: "Well, even if the alternative medicine treatment doesn't actually work, it's just a harmless placebo." The idea of knowingly promoting alternative medicine treatments that don't work beyond the placebo effect unethically embraces an approach to mental health care that encourages deception and ignores the scientific evidence.
"Are clinically proven to work"	Your ears should perk up with this one. The first warning sign with this statement is that no treatments in mental health care are "proven to work" because the scientific methods used to evaluate them can only provide degrees of support, not full-blown proof. People who advertise their treatments as "proven" are unlikely to understand or care about science literacy. The second warning sign is that most science-informed clinicians understand that even evidence-based treatments are imperfect and don't work for everyone.
"Are unknown to science"	This trope capitalizes on the *science of the gaps* fallacy (see page 210), which is often used to promote pseudoscientific approaches that are baseless and implausible. It sounds like, "Science doesn't have all the answers; therefore, we're justified in using this approach." A variant of this trope argues that people are so unique and individualized that current scientific methods are unable to systematically study who might benefit from the approach. These kinds of tropes ignore the fact that the existence of many unanswered scientific questions never justifies the promotion of pseudoscience.
"Aren't in the pocket of Big Pharma"	If I had a Big Pharma check for every time I've been accused on social media of being a Big Pharma shill, then I might actually believe my accusers. Funny enough, the vast majority of clinical psychologists, including myself, do not prescribe medications and have nothing to do with Big Pharma. The thrust of this trope is an attempt to undermine mainstream mental health care by discrediting its capitalist origins (i.e., genesis), thereby committing a *genetic fallacy* (see page 208). Health approaches should be evaluated based on their merit, not whether all mental health professionals are perceived as "paid shills." There are justified reasons to be concerned about the influence of Big Pharma and the biomedical industry on both research and clinical practice that can lead to conflicts of interest, commercialization pressure, biased science, hyped results, and erosion of public confidence in clinicians and health care systems.

Alternative Medicine Tropes "Unlike in mainstream mental health care, alternative medicine treatments . . ."	**Corrections**
	But the evils of Big Pharma aren't solved by the promotion of pseudoscience. It's also important to note the hypocrisy of this trope, which ignores the fact that alternative medicine is driven by the influence of a multi-trillion-dollar wellness industry that we might facetiously call Big Placebo, Big Supplement, or Big Pseudoscience. A popular variant of this trope is the quip "Follow the money." So yes, alternative medicine promoters would like you to follow the money—just not *their* money.
"Aren't allopathic medicine"	If someone promotes a health approach by contrasting it with the term "allopathy" or "allopathic medicine," then it's likely you're about to hear some pseudoscience apologetics. "Allopathy" was coined in 1810 by the inventor of homeopathy, Samuel Hahnemann. The term was used to describe treating a symptom with its opposite, unlike homeopathy, which is in part based on the principle of "like cures like," meaning that a disease can be cured by a substance that produces similar symptoms in healthy people. Nowadays, some consider the terms to be pejorative. "Allopathy" most often refers to the opposite of alternative medicine: mainstream medicine, evidence-based medicine, traditional medicine, conventional medicine, Western medicine, etc.
"Aren't Western medicine"	Science is a process without borders. Medicine isn't Western, Eastern, allopathic, alternative, functional, integrative, etc. Those are marketing terms. There are approaches supported by evidence and ones that aren't. Ironically, many of the most popular alternative medicine treatments were actually developed in "Western" countries—for example, homeopathy (Germany), chiropractic (United States), naturopathy (United States), detoxification diets (United States), ionic foot baths (United States), reflexology ("rediscovered" in the United States), hydrotherapy (Germany), and IV vitamin therapy (United States).
"Have been used for centuries"	This trope commits the *appeal to tradition* fallacy, which argues that an idea promoted in the past is valid by virtue of its historical status. Just because our ancestors used a particular treatment doesn't mean that it's effective. Ironically again, many popular alternative medicine treatments were actually developed relatively recently, including homeopathy (1790s), chiropractic (1890s), naturopathy (1890s), Reiki (first school in 1922), reflexology (1920s), and hydrotherapy (1800s).

Alternative Medicine Tropes "Unlike in mainstream mental health care, alternative medicine treatments . . ."	**Corrections**
"Are natural"	It's peculiar to argue that it's natural to dilute plant products out of existence into a homeopathic remedy or to stick acupuncture needles into one's skin to stimulate the body's "natural self-healing process." This trope commits the *appeal to nature* fallacy—the false belief that what is natural is good—to argue that alternative medicine treatments are better than evidence-based ones. One way to highlight the absurdity of the trope is to point to bad or neutral things that are sometimes also considered natural, such as poison ivy or dirt.
"Are holistic and treat the whole person"	Saying that an approach is holistic doesn't make it so and doesn't transform pseudoscience into evidence-based care. This trope ignores the reality that mainstream mental health care focuses on many interacting aspects of a person's world within a biopsychosocial framework. Practically, this means that competent clinicians listen to their patients and reach out to other regulated health care providers to assist in addressing nutrition, exercise, medication management, interpersonal relationships, psychological and behavioral patterns, etc. Mainstream mental health care is holistic in its foundation, and pseudoscience couldn't be more unholistic.
"Are being suppressed"	If someone is telling you that most scientists and health professionals are suppressing research to keep people mentally unwell and to increase financial earnings, then they're assuming widespread malevolence. At the beginning of Chapter 5, when the Medical Medium stated that "research and medicine stay away from the discussion on toxic heavy metals," he was invoking this conspiratorial trope. Debunking or refusing to implement pseudoscientific treatments is not "suppressing" them or "hiding the truth" no matter how much alternative medicine promoters would like you to believe otherwise.
"Are just as noneffective"	This trope points the finger at mainstream mental health care by suggesting that its treatments lack high-quality evidence to support their use. And it's true: There remains much room to improve our treatments. The solution, however, is better science—not the promotion of more unsupported treatments and pseudoscientific ones that have been thoroughly discredited.

Alternative Medicine Propaganda Tactics

Alternative Medicine Propaganda Tactics	Description
Publishing in pseudoscientific journals	Countless peer-reviewed academic journals exist that range in quality and pseudoscientific features. Studies and ideas that are rejected in popular scientific journals may find a home in ones that promote alternative medicine to lend them a veneer of scientific legitimacy.
Baiting and switching	Promoters of alternative medicine will sometimes deceive and swindle using a bait-and-switch tactic. It involves first baiting with legitimate treatments that are part of evidence-based practice (e.g., discussing a focus on nutrition or exercise in one's treatment plan) and then switching to the promotion of pseudoscientific treatments, such as homeopathy or energy healing.
Use of misleading language	The use of invented, distorted, and misleading language is a classic propaganda tactic. For example, if you peruse websites within the alternative medicine community, you will inevitably stumble upon the term *dis-ease*. Not *disease*, but *dis-ease*, with a hyphen. It's an imprecise term, whereby the hyphen is intended to disempower specific health concerns by reducing their emphasis and instead focus on treating the natural state of *ease* that has been disrupted or imbalanced. Other examples of this tactic include using the term *sick care* in contrast to health care to highlight problems with the mainstream health care system, and using the anti-psychiatry term *neurotoxins* to describe psychiatric medications. On social media, you will also find manipulation of text and font, for example: *$cience*, *Science™*, and *pHARMa*.
Building community	If you hang out enough in alternative medicine online spaces, then you'll become aware of how inclusive, welcoming, validating, and intimate they can feel. Parasocial relationships can develop quickly and involve a sense of closeness to people you don't actually know. Feeling connected to the characters in your favorite television show is an example of a parasocial relationship experience. When members of online communities share personal stories of their mental health journeys and feel bonded to one another, it can become easier to trust the information that is circulated. When communities bond over alternative medicine, the ground can become fertile for sharing misinformation and pseudoscience marketing.

Common Thinking Errors (Cognitive Biases)

Thinking Error	Description
Affect heuristic	Relying on our emotions rather than information to make decisions
Anchoring heuristic	Relying too heavily on the first piece of information we encounter—known as an "anchor"—when making decisions.
Availability heuristic	Relying on information that comes to mind quickly and easily when judging the validity of an idea or making decisions.
Barnum effect	Accepting generic information or vague statements as descriptive of ourselves. Think: horoscopes.
Base rate neglect	Neglecting or ignoring statistical information—known as base rates—in favor of information pertaining to only a specific case about a person or event.
Belief bias	Judging the strength of an argument based on how plausible the conclusion sounds rather than the strength of its premises.
Belief perseverance	Clinging to beliefs despite repeated and overwhelming counterevidence.
Bias blind spot	Believing that it's other people who are prone to cognitive biases while remaining blind to our own. It's a meta-bias: a bias about our biases.
Confirmation bias	Seeking out evidence consistent with our beliefs and denying or distorting evidence that doesn't fit with our beliefs.
Framing effect	Allowing ourselves to be influenced by the way information is presented or "framed" or worded to us rather than the information itself.
Groupthink	Being preoccupied with what the group thinks rather than critical evaluation of the information.
Halo effect	Letting positive impressions of people, brands, products, or services in one area positively influence our thoughts and feelings in other areas.
Hindsight bias	Looking at past events and thinking they were easily predictable.
Illusory correlation	Perceiving a relationship between two events where none exists.
In-group bias	Unfairly favoring those who belong to your own group.
Naïve realism	Believing that the world is precisely as we see it.

Thinking Error	Description
Representativeness heuristic	Estimating the probability of an event based on its similarity to a mental prototype or stereotype.
Sunk cost	The tendency to follow through on an activity because we've already invested time, effort, or resources, regardless of whether the costs of continuing outweigh the benefits.
Survivorship bias	Overlooking failures because they lack visibility and instead basing conclusions only on successes.

Logical Fallacies Used to Promote Alternative Medicine

Logical Fallacy	Description
Appeal to nature	The false belief that what is natural is good. For example, the trope "Alternative medicine treatments are natural."
Appeal to tradition	Occurs when an idea promoted in the past is argued to be valid by virtue of its historical status. For example, the trope "Alternative medicine treatments have been used for centuries; therefore, they work."
Argument from ignorance	The mistake in assuming that because a treatment hasn't been proved not to work, we can assume it's effective. For example, just because the newest mindfulness app hasn't been debunked yet as an effective treatment for cocaine addiction doesn't mean it works.
Bandwagon fallacy	Erroneously assuming that a popular or widely used treatment is effective. Homeopathy is used by millions of people in the United States alone—but it's not effective for any health condition.
Countless counterfeit	An increasing number of anecdotes doesn't strengthen the quality of evidence. Many people can be wrong. This is known as the countless counterfeit fallacy. A million stories from people saying that homeopathy can effectively treat schizophrenia doesn't make it true.
Genetic fallacy	An attempt to undermine an argument by attacking the origin or genesis of the argument. For example, the trope "Unlike in mainstream mental health care, alternative medicine treatments and practitioners aren't in the historical pocket of Big Pharma."
Golden mean	Occurs when it's argued that the truth must be a compromise between two opposing positions. The clinical psychologist Paul Meehl perfectly captured its essence when he quoted the statistician M. G. Kendall: "A friend of mine once remarked to me that if some people asserted the earth rotated from East to West and others that it rotated from West to East, there would always be a few well-meaning citizens to suggest that perhaps there was something to be said for both sides and that maybe it did a little of one and a little of the other; or that the truth probably lay between the extremes and perhaps did not rotate at all."

Logical Fallacy	Description
	Alternative medicine promoters often use this argument to portray the merits of integrative medicine—a rebranding term related to alternative medicine (discussed in Chapter 4)—the premise of which seeks to integrate the best of both alternative and evidence-based medicine. It's an appeal to a false middle ground (recall that "alternative medicine" that is scientifically shown to work is called "medicine"). As the physician Mark Crislip eminently remarked: "If you mix cow pie with apple pie, it doesn't make the cow pie taste better. It makes the apple pie worse."
Motte and bailey	A slippery rhetorical defense of a bad argument used to push an agenda. It occurs when a person combines two positions that share similarities: One is a safe, uncontroversial claim (the *motte*) and the other is a bold, controversial one (the *bailey*). The arguer first advances the controversial position and, when challenged, runs or retreats to the uncontroversial one. For example, first arguing that Reiki is an effective treatment (the *bailey*) and then retreating to the idea that a placebo can help people feel better (the *motte*), or first arguing that alternative medicine is an effective treatment approach for mental disorders (the *bailey*) and then retreating to the fact that nutrition and exercise are important for health (the *motte*).
Moving the goal posts	This is a metaphor describing when an arguer demands that an opponent address more and more points after the initial counterargument has been made. It's a maddening process because the arguer refuses to concede or accept the opponent's argument. For example: *Person 1*: "Homeopathy effectively treats mental disorders." *Person 2*: "That's not true. Even the National Center of Complementary and Integrative Health indicates that there's little evidence to support homeopathy as an effective treatment for any specific health condition." *Person 1*: "Well, that's just because science doesn't have all of the answers." *Person 2*: "It's true that science is an ever-evolving process. But homeopathy is widely considered by medical experts to be a discredited approach to health because it unequivocally violates fundamental principles in pharmacology." *Person 1*: "Well, if homeopathy is just a placebo, then it can't hurt to try it for mental disorders." *Person 2*: "Legitimizing pseudoscience, including homeopathy, is harmful and unethical." Ad nauseam!

Logical Fallacy	Description
Nirvana fallacy	Also known as the *perfect solution* fallacy. It makes an error in assuming that because disciplines, such as clinical psychology or psychiatry, or evidence-based health care more broadly, are imperfect, they should be rejected. The fallacy erroneously presumes that the alternative solution, such as alternative medicine, is superior.
Post hoc ergo propter hoc	Occurs when we believe that because an event occurred first, it must have caused a later event. This fallacy features prominently in beliefs about the effectiveness of alternative medicine treatments. For example, just because someone's depression symptoms went away after receiving Quantum Neurological Reset Therapy doesn't mean that the treatment works. Sometimes people improve despite the treatment they received rather than because of it.
Science of the gaps	This is a play on the *God of the gaps* fallacy that has historically been used to argue for the existence of God. The fallacy is invoked when proponents claim that only the existence of a supernatural entity can explain phenomena currently unexplainable by science. In a similar way, pseudoscience proponents invoke a *science of the gaps* fallacy to justify unsupported claims. For example, the trope "Alternative medicine treatments work but science doesn't have all of the answers just yet."
Strawman fallacy	This is a distortion of an argument that is a weaker and more easily defeated version of the actual argument. For example, when Tom Cruise proclaimed, "There is no such thing as a chemical imbalance" to argue that Brooke Shields shouldn't use antidepressant medications, he was committing a strawman fallacy. Please see the anti-psychiatry tropes on pages 199–200 for more examples.
Tu quoque	Also called *whataboutism* because it's a rhetorical defense that responds by reversing a claim, charging hypocrisy, or raising a different issue. The response is irrelevant to the truth of the claim. For example: *Person 1*: "Pseudoscientific treatments can be harmful." *Person 2*: "What about Big Pharma?!"

Unequivocal Pseudoscientific Treatments

Pseudoscientific Treatment	Description
Ayurveda	A prescientific, belief-based Indian medical system founded on ancient writings that rely on a "natural" and "holistic" approach to physical and mental health.
Biosound therapy	An approach that involves a person sitting in a chair or lying in a bed covered with devices designed to send combinations of vibrations, imagery, and sounds with different beats and timing. Most practitioners claim that it works by changing brain waves and meditative states.
Chelation therapy	A legitimate therapy for heavy metal poisoning and nothing else. It uses chemicals to bind to metals and remove them from the body. One study reported that approximately half a million people in the United States who experience autism spectrum disorders are subjected to it every year due to the false belief that autism is caused by mercury poisoning from thimerosal in vaccines.
Chiropractic	A form of alternative medicine that focuses on the relationship between the body's structure, primarily of the spine and function. Rooted in mystical concepts, chiropractic "subluxations" are scientifically implausible and indefensible despite some modern chiropractors advertising its theory. With the possible exception of back pain, chiropractic spinal manipulation has not been shown to be effective for any health condition, including mental disorders.
Conversion therapy	The practice of attempting to change a person's sexual orientation or gender identity under the flawed assumptions that same-sex attraction or incongruence between biological sex and gender identity are strictly learned behaviors, morally wrong, and indicative of mental illness, and can be changed. Its harm has been well documented, and most major health organizations, including the American Psychiatric Association and the American Psychological Association, have firmly deemed it unethical. It's been criminally banned in Malta, France, Germany, Albania, Mexico, and Canada. In the United States, about half of states have banned it for minors, but it continues to be promoted and implemented.
Energy medicine	Also called "energy healing" or "energy psychology." A set of therapies premised on the belief that "human energy fields" can be manipulated and balanced. Examples: therapeutic touch, Reiki, polarity therapy, cranial-sacral therapy, thought field therapy, emotional freedom techniques.

Pseudoscientific Treatment	Description
Facilitated communication	Wrongfully posits that many severe developmental disorders are caused by motor problems rather than intellectual disabilities. With a keyboard, "facilitators" supposedly help nonverbal individuals communicate by guiding their arm or hand to type out their thoughts. Despite its widespread promotion, research has shown that "facilitators" are the true authors of these messages with little to no conscious awareness of their own deception, not the individuals they're attempting to assist. The deception can be explained by the psychological phenomenon known as the *ideomotor effect*—the same effect that guides a Ouija board—whereby the "facilitator's" thoughts and expectations inadvertently guide a person's arms or hands to the intended letters on the keyboard.
Hyperbaric oxygen therapy	Involves breathing high levels of oxygen in a pressurized chamber. It's a legitimate treatment only for certain medical uses, such as decompression sickness suffered by divers, carbon monoxide poisoning, and enhanced healing of certain wounds like diabetic foot ulcers. It's often advertised as a treatment for mental disorders without any coherent rationale.
Naturopathy	A self-described system of health care that purports to "blend modern scientific knowledge with traditional and natural forms of medicine," with a philosophy "to stimulate the healing power of the body and treat the underlying causes of disease." Examples: acupuncture, homeopathy, orthomolecular medicine, traditional Chinese medicine.
Neurolinguistic programming (NLP)	A popular self-help approach for personal development and the treatment of mental disorders created in the 1970s and still hot today. Despite its name, it really has nothing to do with neuroscience, linguistics, or programming. Based on outdated and factually incorrect ideas about the workings of the brain, it's been widely discredited for its convoluted use of jargon and reliance on anecdotal evidence in the face of extensive research failing to support its assumptions and effectiveness. A modern offshoot of NLP is the Lightning Process, which claims to draw from NLP in addition to other approaches. The National Institute for Health and Care Excellence in the United Kingdom explicitly advises against the use of the Lightning Process in the treatment of chronic fatigue disorder.

Pseudoscientific Treatment	Description
Ozone therapy	An unsupported medical treatment proposed to "detoxify" and "cleanse" by introducing ozone into the body via the vagina, rectum, or injection (i.e., intramuscularly, subcutaneously, or intravenously). Despite this treatment being marketed on some alternative medicine websites as a treatment for mental disorders, the U.S. Food and Drug Administration states that "ozone is a toxic gas with no known useful medical application in specific, adjunctive, or preventive therapy." It can cause serious adverse effects to the central nervous system, heart, and lungs, and has even resulted in death.
Past life regression therapy	Based on the reincarnation hypothesis. Uses hypnosis to address memories and events that an individual went through before they were born in this life.
Scientology's Narconon program	A drug treatment program that avoids the assistance of mental health professionals and promotes unsupported therapy components, such as drug-free withdrawal and megadosing vitamins while sitting in a sauna to sweat out "harmful toxins naturally."

How to Produce a Thought Record

A Thought Record is one specific tool that you can use to start to apply cognitive-behavioral therapy (CBT) principles on your own or in conjunction with a mental health professional. It involves:

- A way to use CBT in everyday life situations
- A way to use a variety of specific CBT strategies
- A way to help regulate emotions and problem-solve
- Five columns: Situation, Emotions, Automatic Thoughts, Rational Responses, Helpful Action. Here's an easy sample template:

Sample Thought Record				
Situation (who, what, when, where?)	**Emotions** (rate 0–10)	**Automatic Thoughts** (what was going through your mind?)	**Rational Responses** (balanced, helpful, realistic thoughts)	**Helpful Action**
Jane is super late picking me up from work.	Angry = 8/10 Anxious = 6/10 Sad = 5/10	I'm angry because Jane only thinks about herself. If she cared about me, then she'd be here.	It's possible that Jane just hit some traffic or something important happened. Just because she's late doesn't mean she doesn't care about me.	I'm going to troubleshoot: First, I'll call Jane and if she doesn't answer, then I'll email. If I don't hear back in 10 minutes, then I'll catch an Uber.
		I'm anxious because I have so many things to do when I get home and now I'll be late.	If I'm late for my dinner date with my friends, that's okay. I can cope—everyone is late sometimes.	I'm going to practice some deep breathing exercises, which I find relaxing.
		My friends are expecting me to meet them for dinner soon, and now they'll be annoyed with me because I'll be late too. I'm sad because my relationship with Jane just isn't what it used to be. It's falling apart.	I might be jumping to conclusions about my relationship with Jane. It's okay to feel sad, but that doesn't necessarily mean that our friendship is on the rocks.	I might have a conversation with Jane tomorrow to hear her side of the story and to express my concerns about our relationship.

Your cue for when to fill out a Thought Record is the experience of an uncomfortable emotion. For instance, if you're feeling anxious, angry, annoyed, sad, etc., go fill one out, either in real time or at the end of the day.

Let's walk through the easy, mundane example above to illustrate the process. Say your friend Jane is late to pick you up from work. The ***Situation*** column is the easiest. You just write down what's happening or what happened. There's no guessing what happened, what someone's thinking, what could happen in the future, etc. It's just objective and there's no interpretation involved: what, who, when, where.

The ***Emotions*** column is descriptive too. It's where you write down all the emotions that you're feeling. Then rate the intensity from 0 to 10, such as "Angry = 8/10, Anxious = 6/10, Sad 5/10."

In the ***Automatic Thoughts*** column, write down whatever springs to mind when thinking about the situation. One helpful tip is to ask yourself why you're feeling the emotions you wrote in the previous column. For example, first ask, "Why am I feeling angry?" and then answer: "I'm feeling angry because Jane only thinks about herself." Continue the process with all the emotions you're experiencing. "I'm anxious because I have so many things to do when I get home and now I'll be late." "I'm sad because my relationship with Jane is falling apart."

Some patients find the ***Rational Responses*** column the most difficult, and it's understandable because it's where we try to peel off those biased lenses. It's where the thought challenging occurs. It's the cognitive work—the "C" in the CBT acronym. The goal is to generate helpful, balanced, realistic thoughts, even if you don't believe them right away. You can use a variety of questions that inspire critical thinking to aid in your endeavor, such as:

- What's the evidence that my automatic thoughts are true? And untrue?
- What's the worst thing that could happen? How about the best and most realistic outcome?
- Could I live through any of it?
- What's another way I could think about this situation?
- Taking a step back, what's the bigger picture?
- What's the probability that this will happen?
- Am I thinking in rigid, all-or-nothing terms?
- What's the gray zone here?
- Is this situation solvable? How so?
- What difference will this make in my life in a week from now? In 1 year? In 10 years?
- What's most important in my life?
- If I talked to someone whose opinion I value, what would they say about this situation?

In addition to broadly brainstorming other ways to think about this situation, you could also use the ***Rational Responses*** column to directly challenge the specific thoughts in your ***Automatic Thoughts*** column. For example, you could challenge the thought "I'm angry because Jane only thinks about herself. If she cared about me, then she'd be here." To challenge this thought, counteract it: "It's possible that Jane just hit some traffic or something important happened. Just because she's late doesn't mean she doesn't care about me."

The last column is ***Helpful Action***. It's the behavioral work—the "B" in the CBT acronym, which can involve participating in pleasurable and effortful activities and finding manageable ways to confront avoidance and anxiety-provoking situations. This column is versatile because it can be used in three ways. First, you could generate behaviors to problem-solve the situation. For instance, you could write: "I'm going to troubleshoot: I'll call her first and if she doesn't answer, then I'll email. If I don't hear back in 10 minutes, then I'll catch an Uber."

Second, you could generate behaviors to manage the uncomfortable emotions from the ***Emotions*** column. For instance, you could write: "I'm going to practice some deep breathing exercises, which I find relaxing."

Third, you could generate what are called *behavioral experiments* to test out the thoughts in the ***Rational Responses*** column. For instance, to test the rational response "It's possible that Jane just hit some traffic," you could write in this column, "I might have a conversation with Jane tomorrow to hear her side of the story." Behavioral experiments are useful because they can help us gather evidence on—and therefore believe—the more helpful ways of thinking that we previously generated.

A Flavor of Evidence-Based Treatments

Evidence-Based Treatment	Description
Acceptance and commitment therapy (ACT)	An approach that incorporates elements of CBT, mindfulness meditation strategies, behavior change strategies, and a focus on what patients value in life. Involves noticing, accepting, and embracing uncomfortable mental experiences and circumstances. Hundreds of RCTs evaluating ACT have been conducted for a range of mental health concerns—its use is most strongly supported for the management of chronic pain, followed by weaker evidence behind its use for the treatment of depressive and anxiety disorders.
Behavioral activation	An advanced branch of CBT for the treatment of depression that focuses on behaviors. Involves finding helpful ways to confront avoidance and increase engagement in both pleasurable and effortful activities.
Cognitive-behavioral therapy (CBT)	Among the most researched and scientifically supported treatments in the world for numerous mental health concerns. Focuses on the connection between thoughts, emotions, and behaviors to challenge how we think and change what we do. Also, an umbrella term for several advanced approaches designed to address specific mental health concerns.

Evidence-Based Treatment	Description
Cognitive processing therapy	An advanced branch of CBT designed for the treatment of posttraumatic stress disorder (PTSD) that focuses on thoughts and beliefs. Initially involves examining the question of why the trauma occurred to increase awareness of how it affects a patient's life and views about themselves, others, and the world. Patients then challenge their thoughts and beliefs in ways that helpfully allow them to make sense of the trauma and heal.
Dialectical behavior therapy (DBT)	An approach designed for the treatment of borderline personality disorder that incorporates elements of CBT, mindfulness meditation, communication skills, emotion regulation skills, and distress tolerance skills. The dialectic in DBT is a fancy term that refers to learning how to hold multiple truths at once about one's experiences. In DBT, we both accept that our experiences are valid and break free from our all-or-none thinking and behaving patterns.
Exposure and response prevention (ERP)	An advanced branch of CBT designed for the treatment of obsessive-compulsive disorder that focuses on behaviors. Involves safely, voluntarily, and gradually exposing oneself to situations that trigger obsessions (i.e., exposure) so that patients can practice refraining from compulsions (i.e., response prevention).
Family therapy	Numerous forms of family therapy have received varying levels of scientific support for the treatment of a range of mental health concerns, particularly for children and adolescents.
Interpersonal therapy	A form of psychotherapy with a strong evidence base for the treatment of depression. Focuses on four major areas: (a) grief and loss; (b) major life transitions, such as job or relationship loss; (c) conflicts in relationships; and (d) problems associated with starting or maintaining relationships.
Motivational interviewing (MI)	A communication style that's been heavily researched and used to address addiction and mental health concerns. It takes an empathic, nonjudgmental approach to conversation that respects another person's autonomy. Helps motivate patients to change behavior by eliciting their own reasons for wanting to change and validating their independence and personal control.

Evidence-Based Treatment	Description
Prolonged exposure	An advanced branch of CBT designed for the treatment of PTSD that focuses on behaviors. Involves repeated voluntarily and safely negotiated exposure to trauma-related thoughts, emotions, memories, and situations to soften the powerful grip of trauma-related distress, avoidance, nightmares, and flashbacks.
Psychiatric medications	A range of different medications are used to treat different mental health concerns, each with varying levels of scientific support compared to placebo. For example, antipsychotics for psychotic disorders; mood stabilizers for bipolar disorders; antidepressants (e.g., selective serotonin reuptake inhibitors) for depressive and anxiety disorders; naltrexone for alcohol use disorders; opioid agonist therapies for opioid use disorders; stimulants for attention-deficit hyperactivity disorder, etc.
Psychodynamic therapy	The modern, updated, scientifically plausible version of Freudian psychoanalysis. Maintains that much of mental life is conflicted, occurs outside of awareness, and can be traced to early life experiences. Clinicians and patients work together to increase awareness of unconscious patterns of thinking and behaving, especially as they show up in the therapeutic relationship. Supported by numerous RCTs, high-quality reviews, and meta-analyses, particularly for depressive disorders, anxiety disorders, and personality disorders.

Acknowledgments

"Writing a book will be fun," I told myself before I started. It was totally fun—and challenging and rewarding. But I underestimated just how green I was to the process. Enter my literary agent, Lucinda Halpern. I can't believe how much I lucked out. She's among the most talented people I've ever met. She's a leader in her craft and I'm eternally grateful that she and her masterful team took a chance on me. She saw my book for what it could be, and it wouldn't exist without her. I may have also inadvertently turned her into a psychologist, as she was tasked with managing my anxiety during every stage of production. Thank you, and sorry.

To all the outstanding people at Penguin Random House Canada, Oxford University Press, and Audible, especially my editors, Craig Pyette and Sarah Harrington, thank you for challenging and bolstering my ideas in a way that finessed their readability.

Timothy Caulfield was my mentor behind the scenes. He saw the desperate need for a book about mental health misinformation and supported me every step of the way during his spare time; frequently checking in, advising, and offering to chat. His encouragement and enthusiasm were so motivating. Thank you, my friend.

Good science communication is like being part of a championship-winning sports team. I've learned from so many diverse expert voices and science communicators over the past several years, each bringing to the table their own unique skill set, many of whom supported this book in various ways. Special thank you to: Candice Basterfield, Derek Beres, Tyler Black, Hannah Blum, Jean Brown, Michelle Cohen, Edzard Ernst, Yves Gagnon, Bernie Garrett, Marvin Goldfried, David Gorski, Jennifer Gunter, Britt Hermes, Annie Hickox, David Hodgins, Peter Hotez, Stephen Hupp, Stanley Kutcher, Ryan Marino, Sulman Mirza, Gordon Pennycook, Brent Phillips, Cyriac Abby Phillips, Joe Pierre, Rina Raphael, and Melanie Trecek-King.

This book would also not be possible without my patients over the years who allowed me the privilege of sharing in their mental health journeys. They opened my eyes to the realities of clinical practice, the devastation of mental illness, and the triumph of human spirit. They also showed me the limits of our knowledge and treatments and inspired me to fight against the exploitation of those limits.

To my former patient Tamara (pseudonym), who I interviewed for this book: "It matters not how strait the gate, how charged with punishments the scroll, I am the master of my fate: I am the captain of my soul. A thousand times, thank you." And a fist bump.

Thank you to everyone on social media who has engaged with my material, enhanced my knowledge, cheerled my mission, and supported me personally. As a result of speaking out against the harms of pseudoscience, I've received a lot of online harassment. I've received death threats, personal attacks, and frivolous complaints to my regulatory body and university. I've been constantly lied about, trolled, and cyberstalked. But during all that commotion, I continue to receive overwhelming support online, effectively drowning it out. Your kindness is seen and appreciated.

Thank you to all my friends and family for their excitement and energy, especially my parents, Heidi and Lou. During my youth, from her hospital bed, cognitively impaired from pain and massive doses of opioids and benzodiazepines, my mother still found a way to help me with my homework and teach me how to write. My father, through it all, taught me everything else.

Lastly, thank you to Leslie. Without her love, I wouldn't have been able to fulfill this dream.

About the Author

Jonathan N. Stea, PhD, RPsych, is a full-time practicing clinical psychologist and an adjunct assistant professor in the Department of Psychology at the University of Calgary. Clinically, he specializes in the assessment and treatment of concurrent addiction and mental disorders. He's a two-time winner of the University of Calgary's Award for Excellence in Clinical Supervision and coeditor of the book *Investigating Clinical Psychology: Pseudoscience, Fringe Science, and Controversies*. Dr. Stea has published extensively as a science communicator, with regular contributions to *Scientific American* and *Psychology Today*, among other outlets, and has appeared on numerous mainstream media television and radio shows, as well as podcasts. He was the 2022 recipient of the John G. Paterson Award from the Psychologists' Association of Alberta, which is an annual award presented for the exceptional contribution to portraying psychological knowledge to the public. Dr. Stea has cultivated a strong social media presence in his quest to expose and protect against mental health misinformation and pseudoscience. You can follow him on X (formerly Twitter), Facebook, and Instagram.

Source Notes

Chapter 1

American Psychiatric Association. (2022). *Diagnostic and statistical manual of mental disorders* (5th ed., text revision).

American Psychological Association. (2019). *Clinical practice guideline for the treatment of depression across three age cohorts*. https://www.apa.org/depression-guideline

Astin, J. A. (1998). Why patients use alternative medicine: Results of a national study. *JAMA*, *279*, 1548–1553.

Bharwani, K. D., Kersten, A. B., Stone, A. L., Birklein, F., Bruehl, S., Dirckx, M., Drummond, P. D., Gierthmuhlen, J., Goebel, A., Knudsen, L., & Huygen, F. J. P. M. (2021). Denying the truth does not change the facts: A systematic analysis of pseudoscientific denial of complex regional pain syndrome. *Journal of Pain Research, 14*, 3359–3376.

Brogan, K. (2016). *A mind of your own: The truth about depression and how women can heal their bodies to reclaim their lives*. Harper Collins Publishers.

Curd, M., & Cover, J. A. (1998). *Philosophy of science: The central issues*. W. W. Norton & Co.

Demyttenaere, K., Bruffaerts, R., Posada-Villa, J., Gasquet, I., Kovess, V., Lepine, J. P., Angermeyer, M. C., Bernert, S., de Girolamo, G., Morosini, P., Polidori, G., Kikkawa, T., Kawakami, N., Ono, Y., Takeshima, T., Uda, H., Karam, E. G., Fayyad, J. A., Karam, A. N. . . . WHO World Mental Health Survey Consortium. (2004). Prevalence, severity, and unmet need for treatment of mental disorders in the World Health Organization World Mental Health Surveys. *JAMA*, *291*, 2581–2590.

Farias, M., Maraldi, E., Wallenkampf, K. C., & Lucchetti, G. (2020). Adverse events in meditation practices and meditation-based therapies: A systematic review. *Acta Psychiatrica Scandinavica, 142*(5), 374–393. doi:10.1111/acps.13225. Epub 2020 Aug 21. PMID: 32820538.

Grand View Research (2023). *Complementary and alternative medicine market size, share & trends analysis report by intervention (botanicals, mind healing, body healing, external energy, sensory healing), by distribution method, and segment forecasts, 2021–2028*. https://www.grandviewresearch.com/industry-analysis/complementary-alternative-medicine-market

Josefson, D. (2001). Rebirthing therapy banned after girl died in 70-minute struggle. *BMJ*, *322*, 1014.

Lilienfeld, S. O. (2007). Psychological treatments that cause harm. *Perspectives on Psychological Science*, *2*, 53–70.

Lilienfeld, S. O. (2015). Introduction to Special Section on Pseudoscience in Psychiatry. *Canadian Journal of Psychiatry*, *60*(12), 531–533.

Lilienfeld, S. O., Lynn, S. J., & Lohr, J. M. (2014). *Science and pseudoscience in clinical psychology*. Guilford Press.

Marinus, J., Moseley, G. L., Birklein, F., Baron, R., Maihofner, C., Kingery, W. S., & van Hilten, J. J. (2011). Clinical features and pathophysiology of complex regional pain syndrome. *The Lancet, Neurology*, *10*, 637–648.

McKay, D., & Jensen-Doss, A. (2021). Harmful treatments in psychotherapy. *Clinical Psychology: Science and Practice*, *28*(1), 2–4.

McNally, R. J. (2003). Is the pseudoscience concept useful for clinical psychology? The demise of pseudoscience. *Scientific Review of Mental Health Practice*, *2*.

Meichenbaum, D., & Lilienfeld, S. O. (2018). How to spot hype in the field of psychotherapy: A 19-item checklist. *Professional Psychology: Research and Practice*, *49*, 22–30.

Mongelli, F., Georgakopoulos, P., & Pato, M. T. (2020). Challenges and opportunities to meet the mental health needs of underserved and disenfranchised populations in the United States. *Journal of Lifelong Learning in Psychiatry*, *18*, 16–24.

National Center for Complementary and Integrative Health. (2023). *"Detoxes" and "cleanses": What you need to know*. https://www.nccih.nih.gov/health/detoxes-and-cleanses-what-you-need-to-know

Norcross, J. C., Koocher, G. P., & Ariele, G. (2006). Discredited psychological treatments and tests: A Delphi poll. *Professional Psychology: Research and Practice*, *37*, 515.

Patel, V., Maj, M., Flisher, A. J., De Silva, M. J., Koschorke, M., Prince, M., & WPA Zonal and Member Society Representatives. (2010). Reducing the treatment gap for mental disorders: A WPA survey. *World Psychiatry*, *9*, 169–176.

Rogan, J. (2020, July 30). *Nancy Panza #1517* [Audio podcast]. Joe Rogan Experience. https://open.spotify.com/episode/01A5ICPmRS5edQeMIB71wn

Sagan, C., & Druyan, A. (1995). *The demon-haunted world: Science as a candle in the dark*. Random House.

Schulz, P., & Hede, V. (2018). Alternative and complementary approaches in psychiatry: Beliefs versus evidence. *Dialogues in Clinical Neuroscience*, *20*, 207–214.

Shattock, M. J., & Tipton, M. J. (2012). "Autonomic conflict": A different way to die during cold water immersion? *Journal of Physiology*, *590*, 3219–3230.

Son, H., Song, H. J., Seo, H-J., Lee, H., Choi, S. M., & Lee, S. (2020). The safety and effectiveness of self-administered coffee enema: A systematic review of case reports. *Medicine*, *99*, e21998.

Tiller, N.B., Sullivan, J. P., & Ekkekakis, P. (2023). Baseless claims and pseudoscience in health and wellness: A call to action for the sports, exercise, and nutrition-science community. *Sports Medicine*, *53*, 1–5.

Touch Stone Essentials. (2023). *Pure Body Extra*. https://thegoodinside.com/shop/product/pure-body-extra-strength

Williams, A. J., Botanov, Y., Kilshaw, R. E., Wong, R. E., & Sakaluk, J. K. (2021). Potentially harmful therapies: A meta-scientific review of evidential value. *Clinical Psychology: Science & Practice*, *28*, 5–18.

Yeung, A., Ng, E., & Abi-Jaoude, E. (2022). TikTok and attention-deficit/hyperactivity disorder: A cross-sectional study of social media content quality. *Canadian Journal of Psychiatry*, *67*, 899–906.

Chapter 2

Al-Yateem, N., Rossiter, R. C., Robb, W. F., Slewa-Younan, S. (2018). Mental health literacy of school nurses in the United Arab Emirates. *International Journal of Mental Health Systems*, *12*, 6.

American Psychiatric Association. (2021). *Practice guidelines for the treatment of patients with schizophrenia* (3rd ed.).

American Psychiatric Association. (2022). *Diagnostic and statistical manual of mental disorders* (5th ed., text revision).

American Psychiatric Association. (2023). *Stigma, prejudice, and discrimination against people with mental illness.* https://www.psychiatry.org/patients-families/stigma-and-discrimination

Bahji, A., Socias, M. E., & Bach, P. (2023). Cases: Multiorgan failure in a 38-year-old man with recent consumption of kratom, an atypical opioid. *Psychiatry Research Case Reports, 2,* 100088.

Bandura, A. (2010). Self-efficacy. In I. B. Weiner & W. E. Craighead (Eds.), *The Corsini encyclopedia of psychology* (4th ed., pp. 1534–1536). John Wiley & Sons.

Blum, H. (2020). *The wellness movement's shaming of people with mental illness.* https://halfway2hannah.com/2020/04/16/the-wellness-movements-shaming-of-people-with-mental-illness-and-how-we-come-together/

Bonabi, H., Muller, M., Ajdacic-Gross, V., Eisele, J., Rodgers, S., Seifritz, E., Rossler, W., & Rusch, N. (2016). Mental health literacy, attitudes to help seeking, and perceived need as predictors of mental health service use: A longitudinal study. *Journal of Nervous and Mental Disease, 204,* 321–324.

Breggin, P. (2018). *What should we really call psychiatric drugs?* Mad in America. https://www.madinamerica.com/2018/01/what-really-call-psychiatric-drugs/

Byrne, R. (2006). *The secret.* Atria Books.

Caulfield, T. (2018). *Vaccines, public trust and learning from my hate mail.* Policy Options. https://policyoptions.irpp.org/magazines/november-2018/vaccines-public-trust-and-learning-from-my-hate-mail/

Cavojova, V., Srol, J. & Bolova Mikuskova, E. (2022). How scientific reasoning correlates with health-related beliefs and behaviors during the COVID-19 pandemic? *Journal of Health Psychology, 27,* 534–547.

Centers for Disease Control and Prevention. (2022). *Vaccine effectiveness: How well do flu vaccines work?* https://www.cdc.gov/flu/vaccines-work/vaccineeffect.htm

Chao, L. L. (2019). Improvements in Gulf War Illness symptoms after near-infrared transcranial and intranasal photobiomodulation: Two case reports. *Military Medicine, 184*(9/10), 5.

Club Random with Bill Maher. (2023, June 25). *Robert F. Kennedy Jr.* https://www.youtube.com/watch?v=V0dQD1Z6j60

CNN Larry King Live. (2005, December 15). *Interview with Bill Maher.* Transcript retrieved from https://transcripts.cnn.com/show/lkl/date/2005-12-15/segment/01

Dong, C., Shi, H., Liu, P., Si, G., & Yan, Z. (2022). A critical overview of systematic reviews and meta-analyses of light therapy for non-seasonal depression. *Psychiatry Research, 314,* 114686.

Ellis, J., Mullan, J., Worsley, A., & Pai, N. (2012). The role of health literacy and social networks in arthritis patients' health information-seeking behavior: A qualitative study. *International Journal of Family Medicine, 1,* 1–6.

Elyamani, R., & Hammoud, H. (2020). Mental health literacy of healthcare providers in Arab Gulf countries: A systematic review. *Journal of Primary Care & Community Health, 11,* 2150132720972271.

Foa, E. B., & McLean, C. P. (2016). The efficacy of exposure therapy for anxiety-related disorders and its underlying mechanisms: The case of OCD and PTSD. *Annual Review of Clinical Psychology, 12,* 1–28.

Gorski, D. (2012). *Luc Montagnier and the Nobel Disease.* Science-Based Medicine. https://sciencebasedmedicine.org/luc-montagnier-and-the-nobel-disease/

Gorski, D. (2021). *Germ theory denial in the age of the Covid-19 pandemic.* Science-Based Medicine. https://sciencebasedmedicine.org/germ-theory-denial-in-the-age-of-the-covid-19-pandemic/

Government of Canada. (2018). *Unauthorized "Saj" kratom products seized from two Edmonton stores may pose serious health risks.* https://recalls-rappels.canada.ca/en/alert-recall/unauthorized-saj-kratom-products-seized-two-edmonton-stores-may-pose-serious-health

Hao, Y., Wu, Q., Luo, X., Chen, S., Qi, C., Long, J., Xiong, Y., Liao, Y., & Liu, T. (2020). Mental health literacy of non-mental health nurses: A mental health survey in four general hospitals in Hunan Province, China. *Frontiers in Psychiatry, 11*, 507969.

Jayanti, R., & Burns, A. (1998). The antecedents of preventive health care behavior: An empirical study. *Journal of the Academy of Marketing Science, 26*, 6–15.

Kilincel, S., & Muratdagi, G. (2021). Knowledge and awareness level of mental health literacy among pediatricians. *Annals of Clinical and Analytical Medicine, 12*, 532–536.

Koran, L. M., & Simpson, H. B. (2013). *Practice guideline for the treatment of patients with obsessive-compulsive disorder.* American Psychiatric Association. https://psychiatryonline.org/pb/assets/raw/sitewide/practice_guidelines/guidelines/ocd-watch-1410457187510.pdf

Kutcher, S., Wei, Y., & Coniglio, C. (2016). Mental health literacy: Past, present, and future. *Canadian Journal of Psychiatry, 61*, 154–158.

Lacroix, E., Dobson, K. S., & von Ranson, K. M. (2018). Scope and ethics of psychologists' use of client testimonials on professional websites. *Canadian Psychology, 59*, 232–238.

Landrum, A. R., & Olshansky, A. (2019). The role of conspiracy mentality in denial of science and susceptibility to viral deception about science. *Politics and the Life Sciences, 38*, 193–209.

Light, N., Fernback, P. M., Rabb, N., Geana, M. V., & Sloman, S. A. (2022). Knowledge overconfidence is associated with anti-consensus views on controversial scientific issues. *Science Advances, 8*, 29.

Manchester, K. L. (2007). Louis Pasteur, fermentation, and a rival. *South African Journal of Science, 103*, 377–380.

Matute, H., Yarritu, I., & Vadillo, M. A. (2011). Illusions of causality at the heart of pseudoscience. *British Journal of Psychology, 102*, 392–405.

McCaffrey, E., Chang, S., Farrelly, G., Rahman, A., & Cawthorpe, D. (2017). Mental health literacy in primary care: Canadian Research and Education for the Advancement of Child Health (CanREACH). *Evidence-Based Medicine, 22*, 123–131.

McKay, D., Abramowitz, J. S., & Storch, E. A. (2021). Mechanisms of harmful treatments for obsessive–compulsive disorder. *Clinical Psychology: Science and Practice, 28*, 52–59.

Mendenhall, A. N., & Frauenholtz, S. (2013). Mental health literacy: Social work's role in improving public mental health. *Social Work, 58*(4), 365–368.

Murad, M. H., Asi, N., Alsawas, M., & Alahdab, F. (2016). New evidence pyramid. *BMJ Evidence-Based Medicine, 21*, 125–127.

National Academies of Sciences, Engineering, and Medicine. (2016). *Science literacy: Concepts, contexts, and consequences.* National Academies Press. https://www.chemconnections.org/Reading/Scientific%20Literacy%20NAS%2023595.pdf

National Center for Complementary and Integrative Health. (2022). *Kratom.* https://www.nccih.nih.gov/health/kratom

National Science Board. (2018). *Science and engineering indicators 2018*. NSB-2018-1. National Science Foundation. https://www.nsf.gov/statistics/indicators/

Orenstein, W. A., & Ahmed, R. (2017). Simply put: Vaccination saves lives. *Proceedings of the National Academy of Sciences of the United States of America, 114*, 4031–4033.

Oztas, B., & Aydogan, A. (2021). Assessment of mental health literacy of health professionals. *Journal of Psychiatric Nursing, 12*(3), 198–204.

Piejka, A., & Okruszek, Ł. (2020). Do you believe what you have been told? Morality and scientific literacy as predictors of pseudoscience susceptibility. *Applied Cognitive Psychology, 34*, 1072–1082.

Pierre, J. (2012). Mental illness and mental health: Is the glass half empty or half full? *Canadian Journal of Psychiatry, 57*, 651–658.

Rozenblit, L., & Keil, F. (2002). The misunderstood limits of folk science: An illusion of explanatory depth. *Cognitive Science, 26*, 521–562.

Sagan, C., & Druyan, A. (1995). *The demon-haunted world: Science as a candle in the dark*. Random House.

Schmaltz, R., & Lilienfeld, S. O. (2014). Hauntings, homeopathy, and the Hopkinsville Goblins: Using pseudoscience to teach scientific thinking. *Frontiers in Psychology, 5*, Article 336.

Tambling, R. R., D'Aniello, C., & Russell, B. S. (2021). Mental health literacy: A critical target for narrowing racial disparities in behavioral health. *International Journal of Mental Health and Addiction*, 1–15.

The Decision Lab. (2022). *Why do we think we understand the world more than we actually do?* https://thedecisionlab.com/biases/the-illusion-of-explanatory-depth

The Joe Rogan Experience. (2022). *Episode 1804—Bill Maher*. https://open.spotify.com/episode/2e4JenTP3prIyddkZbLjbR

The Lancet. (2022). Managing the opioid crisis in North America and beyond. *Lancet, 399*(10324), 495.

Thompson-Hollands, J., Farchione, T. J., & Barlow, D. H. (2013). Thought-action fusion across anxiety disorder diagnoses: Specificity and treatment effects. *Journal of Nervous and Mental Disease, 201*, 407–413. https://doi.org/10.1097/NMD.0b013e31828e102c

Vielight. (2023). *Light therapy treatment—research journey*. https://www.vielight.com/light-therapy-treatment-research-journey/

Weiss, S. T., & Douglas, H. E. (2021). Treatment of kratom withdrawal and dependence with buprenorphine/naloxone: A case series and systematic literature review. *Journal of Addiction Medicine, 15*, 167–172.

World Health Organization. (2013). *Health literacy: The solid facts*. WHO Regional Office for Europe.

World Health Organization. (2022). *Safety of Covid-19 vaccines*. https://www.who.int/news-room/feature-stories/detail/safety-of-covid-19-vaccines

World Health Organization. (2022). *Vaccines and immunization*. https://www.who.int/health-topics/vaccines-and-immunization#tab=tab_1

Wu, Q., Luo, X., Chen, S., Qi, C., Long, J., Xiong, Y., Liao, Y., & Liu, T. (2017). Mental health literacy survey of non-mental health professionals in six general hospitals in Hunan Province of China. *PLOS One, 12*, e0180327.

Youngstedt, S. D., Kline, C. E., Reynolds, A. M., Crowley, S. K., Burch, J. B., Khan, N., & Han, S. (2022). Bright light treatment of combat-related PTSD: A randomized controlled trial. *Military Medicine, 187*, e435–e444.

Chapter 3

American Psychiatric Association. (2022). *Diagnostic and statistical manual of mental disorders* (5th ed., text revision).

American Psychological Association. (2019). *Clinical practice guideline for the treatment of depression across three age cohorts.* https://www.apa.org/depression-guideline

Azevedo, F. A., Carvalho, L. R., Grinberg, L. T., Farfel, J. M., Ferretti, R. E., Leite, R. E., Jacob Filho, W., Lent, R., & Herculano-Houzel, S. (2009). Equal numbers of neuronal and nonneuronal cells make the human brain an isometrically scaled-up primate brain. *Journal of Comparative Neurology, 513*, 532–541.

Buchanan-Barker, P., & Barker, P. (2009). The convenient myth of Thomas Szasz. *Journal of Psychiatric and Mental Health Nursing, 16*, 87–98.

CBC News. (2020). *U of O students denounce anti-psychiatry exhibit.* https://www.cbc.ca/news/canada/ottawa/uottawa-psychiatry-protest-1.5443534

Fitelson, E., Kim, S., Baker, A. S., & Leight, K. (2010). Treatment of postpartum depression: Clinical, psychological and pharmacological options. *International Journal of Women's Health, 3*, 1–14.

Hall, H. (2015). *Scientology's war on medicine.* Science-Based Medicine. https://sciencebasedmedicine.org/scientologys-war-on-medicine/

Haslam, N., Tse, J. S. Y., & De Deyne, S. (2021). Concept creep and psychiatrization. *Frontiers in Sociology, 6*, 806147.

Hemens, A. (2000). *Students protest Scientology linked anti-psychiatry exhibit at U of O.* https://thefulcrum.ca/news/students-protest-scientology-linked-anti-psychiatry-exhibit-at-u-of-o/

Hickox, A. (2019). *Are you okay?* The Psychologist. https://www.bps.org.uk/psychologist/are-you-okay

Hickox, A. (2020). *The threat is coming from inside the house.* The Psychologist. https://www.bps.org.uk/psychologist/threat-coming-inside-house

Kent, S. A., & Manca, T. A. (2014). A war over mental health professionalism: Scientology versus psychiatry. *Mental Health, Religion & Culture, 17*, 1–23.

Kho, K. H., van Vreeswijk, M. F., Simpson, S., & Zwinderman, A. H. (2003). A meta-analysis of electroconvulsive therapy efficacy in depression. *Journal of ECT, 19*, 139–147.

Lindblad, L., Nordenskjold, A., Otterbeck, A., & Nordenskjold, A. M. (2022). Risk factors for mortality of medical causes within 30 days of electroconvulsive therapy. *Journal of Affective Disorders, 320*, 527–533.

López-Muñoz, F., & Alamo, C. (2009). Monoaminergic neurotransmission: The history of the discovery of antidepressants from 1950s until today. *Current Pharmaceutical Design, 15*, 1563–1586.

McNally, R. J. (2021). Network analysis of psychopathology: Controversies and challenges. *Annual Review of Clinical Psychology, 17*, 31–53.

Neill, U. S. (2005). Tom Cruise is dangerous and irresponsible. *Journal of Clinical Investigation, 115*, 1964–1965.

Nonprofit Explorer. (2022). *Tax filings per year for Citizens Commission on Human Rights.* https://projects.propublica.org/nonprofits/organizations/680005541

Patel, K., Allen, S., Haque, M. N., Angelescu, I., Baumeister, D., & Tracy, D. K. (2016). Bupropion: A systematic review and meta-analysis of effectiveness as an antidepressant. *Therapeutic Advances in Psychopharmacology, 6,* 99–144.

Pierre, J. (2012). Mental illness and mental health: Is the glass half empty or half full? *Canadian Journal of Psychiatry, 57,* 651–658.

Pierre, J. M. (2010). The borders of mental disorder in psychiatry and the DSM: Past, present, and future. *Journal of Psychiatric Practice, 16,* 375–386.

Raskin, J. D., Maynard, D., & Gayle, M. C. (2022). Psychologist attitudes toward DSM-5 and its alternatives. *Professional Psychology: Research and Practice, 53,* 553–563.

Ray, L. A., & Grodin, E. N. (2021). Clinical neuroscience of addiction: What clinical psychologists need to know and why. *Annual Review of Clinical Psychology, 17,* 465–493.

Remini, L. (2015). *Troublemaker: Surviving Hollywood and Scientology.* Random House Publishing Group.

Rissmiller, D. J., & Rissmiller, J. H. (2006). Evolution of the antipsychiatry movement into mental health consumerism. *Psychiatric Services (Washington, D.C.), 57*(6), 863–866.

Shields, B. (2005). War of words. *New York Times.* https://www.nytimes.com/2005/07/01/opinion/war-of-words.html

Shorter, E. (2015). The history of nosology and the rise of the Diagnostic and Statistical Manual of Mental Disorders. *Dialogues in Clinical Neuroscience, 17,* 59–67.

Stea, J. N., Black, T. R., & Pierre, J. (2020). *Why anti-psychiatry now fails and harms—formerly a healthy corrective, movement now distracts from real problems and actively hurts people.* MedPage Today. https://www.medpagetoday.com/psychiatry/generalpsychiatry/88526

Surís, A., Holliday, R., & North, C. S. (2016). The evolution of the classification of psychiatric disorders. *Behavioral Sciences (Basel, Switzerland), 6,* 5.

Szasz, T. S. (1960). The myth of mental illness. *American Psychologist, 15,* 113–118.

Szasz, T. S. (1996). *The meaning of mind: Language, morality and neuroscience.* Praeger.

UK ECT Review Group. (2003). Efficacy and safety of electroconvulsive therapy in depressive disorders: A systematic review and meta-analysis. *Lancet, 361,* 799–808.

Verbeeck, W., Bekkering, G. E., Van den Noortgate, W., & Kramers, C. (2017). Bupropion for attention deficit hyperactivity disorder (ADHD) in adults. *Cochrane Database of Systematic Reviews, 10,* CD009504.

Whitley, R. (2012). The antipsychiatry movement: Dead, diminishing, or developing? *Psychiatric Services (Washington, D.C.), 63,* 1039–1041.

Wightman, D. S., Foster, V. J., Krishen, A., Richard, N. E., & Modell, J. G. (2010). Meta-analysis of suicidality in placebo-controlled clinical trials of adults taking bupropion. *Primary Care Companion to the Journal of Clinical Psychiatry, 12,* PCC.09m00894.

Wolraich, M. L., Hagan, J. F., Jr., Allan, C., Chan, E., Davison, D., Earls, M., Evans, S., W., Flinn, S. K., Froehlich, T., Frost, J., Holbrook, J. R., Lehmann, C. U., Lessin, H. R., Okechukwu, K., Pierce, K. L., Winner, J. D., Zurhellen, W., & Subcommittee on Children and Adolescents with Attention-Deficit/Hyperactive Disorder. (2019). Clinical practice guideline for the diagnosis, evaluation, and treatment of attention-deficit/hyperactivity disorder in children and adolescents. *Pediatrics, 144,* e20192528.

Zimmerman, M., & Galione, J. (2010). Psychiatrists' and nonpsychiatrist physicians' reported use of the DSM-IV criteria for major depressive disorder. *Journal of Clinical Psychiatry, 71,* 235–238.

Chapter 4

Bailey, Z. D., Kriger, N., Agenor, M., Graves, J., Linos, N., & Bassett, M. T. (2017). Structural racism and health inequities in the USA: Evidence and interventions. *Lancet*, *389*, 1453–1463.

Beck, A. H. (2004). The Flexner Report and the standardization of American medical education. *JAMA*, *291*, 2139–2140.

Beres, D., Remski, M., & Walker, J. (2023). *Conspirituality: How New Age conspiracy theories became a health threat*. Random House Canada.

Blei, D. (2017). *The false promises of wellness culture*. JSTOR Daily. https://daily.jstor.org/the-false-promises-of-wellness-culture/

Browne, M., Thomson, P., Rockloff, M. J., & Pennycook, G. (2015). Going against the herd: Psychological and cultural factors underlying the "vaccination confidence gap." *PLOS One*, *10*, e0132562.

Bystritsky, A., Hovav, S., Sherbourne, C., Stein, M. B., Rose, R. D., Campbell-Sills, L., Golinelli, D., Sullivan, G., Craske, M. G., & Roy-Byrne, P. P. (2012). Use of complementary and alternative medicine in a large sample of anxiety patients. *Psychosomatics*, *53*, 266–272.

Carlson, P. (2018). *Putting the "fad" in Macfadden*. History. https://www.historynet.com/putting-fad-macfadden/

Caulfield, T. (2012). Commentary: The law, unproven CAM and the two-hats fallacy. *Focus on Alternative and Complementary Therapies*, *17*, 4–8.

Caulfield, T., Marcon, A. R., & Mrudoch, B. (2017). Injecting doubt: Responding to the naturopathic anti-vaccination rhetoric. *Journal of Law and the Biosciences*, *4*, 229–249.

Cohen, M. (2021). *Being healthy is not the same as being virtuous. Illness and disability are not ways to measure the value of a human life*. Medium. https://elemental.medium.com/being-healthy-is-not-the-same-as-being-virtuous-f1d3444c1b2c

Cohen, M. (2022). *"Violating nature's health laws": How an eccentric early 20th century influencer set the stage of the COVID infodemic*. Healthy Debate. https://healthydebate.ca/2022/10/topic/influencer-infodemic-covid/

de Jonge, P., Wardenaar, K. J., Hoenders, H. R., Evans-Lacko, S., Kovess-Masfety, V., Aguilar-Gaxiola, S., Al-Hamzawi, A., Alonso, J., Andrade, L. H., Benjet, C., Bromet, E. J., Bruffaerts, R., Bunting, B., Caldas-de-Almeida, J. M., Dinolova, R. V., Florescu, S., de Girolama, G., Gureje, O., Haro, J. M., . . . Thornicroft, G. (2018). Complementary and alternative medicine contacts by persons with mental disorders in 25 countries: Results from the world mental health surveys. *Epidemiology and Psychiatric Sciences*, *27*, 552–567.

Derkatch, C. (2022). *Why wellness sells: Natural health in a pharmaceutical culture*. John Hopkins University Press.

Duffy, T. P. (2011). The Flexner Report—100 years later. *Yale Journal of Biology and Medicine*, *84*, 269–276.

Dunn, H. L. (1959). What high-level wellness means. *Canadian Journal of Public Health*, *50*, 447–457.

Fontana, R. J., Liou, I., Reuben, A., Suzuki, A., Fiel, M. I., Lee, W., & Navarro, V. (2023). AASLD practice guidance on drug, herbal, and dietary supplement-induced liver injury. *Hepatology*, *77*, 1036–1065.

Global Wellness Institute. (2024). *The 2023 global wellness economy monitor: The leading authority on the wellness economy.* https://globalwellnessinstitute.org/the-2023-global-wellness-economy-monitor/

Gorski, D. (2016). *Functional medicine: The ultimate misnomer in the world of integrative medicine.* Science-Based Medicine. https://sciencebasedmedicine.org/functional-medicine-the-ultimate-misnomer-in-the-world-of-integrative-medicine/

Gorski, D. H., & Novella, S. P. (2014). Clinical trials of integrative medicine: Testing whether magic works? *Trends in Molecular Medicine, 20,* 473–476.

Grand View Research (2023). *Complementary and alternative medicine market size, share & trends analysis report by intervention (botanicals, mind healing, body healing, external energy, sensory healing), by distribution method, and segment forecasts, 2021–2028.* https://www.grandviewresearch.com/industry-analysis/complementary-alternative-medicine-market

Hornsey, M. J., Harris, E. A., & Fielding, K. S. (2018). The psychological roots of anti-vaccination attitudes: A 24-nation investigation. *Health Psychology, 37,* 307–315.

Hyman, M. (2009). *The UltraMind solution: Fix your broken brain by healing your body first: The simple way to defeat depression, overcome anxiety, and sharpen your mind.* Scribner.

Kellogg, J. H. (1883). *Ladies' guide in health and disease: Girlhood, maidenhood, wifehood, motherhood.* W. D. Condit & Co.

Kelly, K. (2022). *American detox: The myth of wellness and how we can truly heal.* North Atlantic Books.

Lindsay, B. (2022). *Naturopaths "not bound by science," lawyer argues in B.C. hearing on fecal transplants for autism.* CBC. https://www.cbc.ca/news/canada/british-columbia/bc-naturopath-fecal-transplants-jason-klop-court-hearing-1.6504615

MacFarlane, D., Hurlstone, M. J., & Ecker, U. K. H. (2020). Protecting consumers from fraudulent health claims: A taxonomy of psychological drivers, interventions, barriers, and treatments. *Social Science & Medicine, 259,* 112790.

Manjoo, F. (2022). Alex Jones and the wellness-conspiracy industrial complex. *New York Times.* https://www.nytimes.com/2022/08/11/opinion/alex-jones-wellness-conspiracy.html

Markel, H. (2017). *The Kelloggs: The battling brothers of Battle Creek.* Pantheon Books.

Marsh, T. N., Coholic, D., Cote-Meek, S., & Najavits, L. M. (2015). Blending Aboriginal and Western healing methods to treat intergenerational trauma with substance use disorder in Aboriginal peoples who live in Northeastern Ontario, Canada. *Harm Reduction Journal, 12,* 14.

Mensah, M., Ogbu-Nwobodo, L., & Shim, R. S. (2021). Racism and mental health equity: History repeating itself. *Psychiatric Services, 72,* 1091–1094.

Mikulic, M. (2022). *Global pharmaceutical industry—statistics and facts.* Statista. https://www.statista.com/topics/1764/global-pharmaceutical-industry/#topicOverview

Mikulic, M. (2023). *Estimated alternative medicine industry revenue in the U. S. from 2013 to 2023.* Statista. https://www.statista.com/statistics/203972/alternative-medicine-revenue-growth/

National Center for Complementary and Integrative Health. (2021). *Homeopathy: What you need to know.* https://www.nccih.nih.gov/health/homeopathy

Raphael, R. (2022). *The gospel of wellness: Gyms, gurus, and the false promise of self-care.* Henry Holt and Co.

Sue, S., Zane, N., Nagayama Hall, G. C., & Berger, L. K. (2009). The case for cultural competency in psychotherapeutic interventions. *Annual Review of Psychology, 60*, 525–548.

Summer, A. (2015). *Will a name change make NIH research center less controversial?* American Association for the Advancement of Science. https://www.aaas.org/will-name-change-make-nih-research-center-less-controversial

Wemrell, M., Olsson, A., & Landgren, K. (2020). The use of complementary and alternative medicine (CAM) in psychiatric units in Sweden. *Issues in Mental Health Nursing, 41*, 946–957.

Whorton, J. C. (2001). From cultism to CAM: The Flexner Report reconsidered. *Complementary Health Practice Review, 6*, 113–125.

Whorton, J. C. (2002). *Nature cures: The history of alternative medicine in America.* Oxford University Press.

Zussman, R. (2022). *Naturopaths, chiropractors have lowest vaccination rates in B.C., officials say.* Global News. https://globalnews.ca/news/8824163/vaccination-rate-bc-health-workers-may-10-2022/

Chapter 5

Benedict, C. (2020). Scott Lilienfeld, psychologist who questioned psychology, dies at 59. *New York Times.* https://www.nytimes.com/2020/10/16/science/scott-lilienfeld-dead.html

Beyerstein, B. L. (n.d.). *Evidence counts: What counts as evidence? A crash course on skepticism and the paranormal.* https://www.skeptic.ca/Skeptics_Tool_Kit.pdf

Colter, W., & Mills, P. J. (2020). Assessing the accuracy of medical intuition: A subjective and exploratory study. *Journal of Alternative and Complementary Medicine (New York, N.Y.), 26*, 1130–1135.

Delgado-López, P. D., & Corrales-García, E. M. (2018). Influence of internet and social media in the promotion of alternative oncology, cancer quackery, and the predatory publishing phenomenon. *Cureus, 10*(5), e2617.

Ernst, E. (2020). *Don't believe what you think: Arguments for and against SCAM.* Imprint Academic Ltd.

Goode, E. (2004). Defying psychiatric wisdom, these skeptics say "prove it." *New York Times.* https://www.nytimes.com/2004/03/09/health/defying-psychiatric-wisdom-these-skeptics-say-prove-it.html

Greenwood, T. A. (2020). Creativity and bipolar disorder: A shared genetic vulnerability. *Annual Review of Clinical Psychology, 16*, 239–264.

Grimes, D. R. (2012). Proposed mechanisms for homeopathy are physically impossible. *Focus on Alternative and Complementary Therapies, 17*, 149–155.

Hitchens, C. (2007). *God is not great: How religion poisons everything.* Twelve.

Ioannidis, J. P. A., Boyack, K. W., & Baas, J. (2020). Updated science-wide author databases of standardized citation indicators. *PLOS Biology, 18*(10), e3000918.

Irmak, M. K. (2014). Schizophrenia or possession? *Journal of Religion and Health, 53*, 773–777.

Kuntz, M. (2012). The postmodern assault on science. If all truths are equal, who cares what science has to say? *EMBO Reports, 13*, 885–889.

Lakatos, I. (1998). Science and pseudoscience. In M. Curd & J. A. Cover (Eds.), *Philosophy of science: The central issues* (pp. 20–26). W. W. Norton & Co.

Lilienfeld, S. O. (2005). *The 10 commandments of helping students distinguish science from pseudoscience in psychology*. APS Observer. https://www.psychologicalscience.org/observer/the-10-commandments-of-helping-students-distinguish-science-from-pseudoscience-in-psychology

Lilienfeld, S. O., et al. (2014). *Science and pseudoscience in clinical psychology*. Guilford Press.

Machado, D., Hicks, O., & Dozois, J. A. (2024). Historical roots in pseudoscience: The importance of intellectual humility. In J. N. Stea & S. Hupp (Eds.), *Investigating clinical psychology: Pseudoscience, fringe science, and controversies* (pp. 13–26). Routledge.

McNally, R. J. (2003). The demise of pseudoscience. *The Scientific Review of Mental Health Practice: Objective Investigations of Controversial and Unorthodox Claims in Clinical Psychology, Psychiatry, and Social Work, 2*, 97–101.

Murdoch, B., Zarzeczny, A., & Caulfield, T. (2018). Exploiting science? A systematic analysis of complementary and alternative medicine clinic websites' marketing of stem cell therapies. *BMJ Open, 8*, e019414.

Prousky, J. E. (2018). Repositioning individualized homeopathy as a psychotherapeutic technique with resolvable ethical dilemmas. *Journal of Evidence-Based Integrative Medicine, 23*.

Radin, D., Hayseen, G., Emoto, M., & Kizu, T. (2006). Double-blind test of the effects of distant intention on water crystal formation. *Explore (New York, N.Y.), 2*, 408–411.

Ross, C. L. (2019). Energy medicine: Current status and future perspectives. *Global Advances in Health and Medicine, 8*. (Retraction published on April 13, 2021)

Rubik, B., Brooks, A. J., & Schwartz, G. E. (2006). In vitro effect of Reiki treatment on bacterial cultures: Role of experimental context and practitioner well-being. *Journal of Alternative and Complementary Medicine, 12*, 7–13.

Schmaltz, R., & Lilienfeld, S. O. (2014). Hauntings, homeopathy, and the Hopkinsville Goblins: Using pseudoscience to teach scientific thinking. *Frontiers in Psychology, 5*, Article 336.

Solzhenitsyn, A. (1973). *The Gulag archipelago*. Harper & Row.

Tajadini, H., Zangiabadi, N., Divsalar, K., Safizadeh, H., Esmaili, Z., & Rafiei, H. (2017). Effect of prayer on intensity of migraine headache: A randomized clinical trial. *Journal of Evidence-Based Complementary & Alternative Medicine, 22*, 37–40.

Trecek-King, M. (2022). How to sell pseudoscience. *Skeptical Inquirer, 46*, 5. https://skepticalinquirer.org/2022/08/how-to-sell-pseudoscience/

William, A. (2015). *Medical Medium: Secrets behind chronic and mystery illness and how to finally heal*. Hay House.

William, A. (2022). *Medical Medium brain saver: Answers to brain inflammation, mental health, OCD, brain fog, neurological symptoms, addiction, anxiety, depression, heavy metals, Epstein-Barr virus*. Hay House.

Wilson, J. A. (2018). Reducing pseudoscientific and paranormal beliefs in university students through a course in science and critical thinking. *Science & Education, 27*, 183–210.

Chapter 6

All That's Interesting. (2018). *Meet Braco—the "healer" who makes people feel better by staring at them*. https://allthatsinteresting.com/braco

Bensley, D. A., Lilienfeld, S. O., Rowan, K., Masciocchi, C. M., & Grain, F. (2019). The generality of belief in unsubstantiated claims. *Applied Cognitive Psychology, 34*, 16–28.

Brown, G., & Brown, J. (2020). *This sweet life: How we lived after Kirby died.* Three Tomatoes Publishing.

Byrne, R. (2006). *The secret.* Atria Books.

CNN Larry King Live. (2006, November 16). *Interview with James Arthur Ray.* Transcript retrieved from http://edition.cnn.com/TRANSCRIPTS/0611/16/lkl.01.html

Crislip, M. (2012). *Perpetual motion: More on the Bravewell Report.* https://sciencebasedmedicine.org/perpetual-motion-more-on-the-bravewell-report/

Douglas, K. M., Uscinski, J. E., Sutton, R. M., Cichocka, A., Nefes, T., Ang, C. S., & Deravi, F. (2019). Understanding conspiracy theories. *Political Psychology, 40*, 3–35.

Kahneman, D. (2011). *Thinking, fast and slow.* Farrar, Strauss, & Giroux.

Kellerman, J., Lewis, J., & Laird, J. D. (1989). Looking and loving: The effects of mutual gaze on feelings of romantic love. *Journal of Research in Personality, 23*, 145–161.

Lilienfeld, S. O., Ammirati, R., & David, M. (2012). Distinguishing science from pseudoscience in school psychology: Science and scientific thinking as safeguards against human error. *Journal of School Psychology, 50*, 7–36.

Lilienfeld, S. O., & Basterfield, C. (2020). The jigsaw puzzle of fraudulent health claims: Missing psychological pieces. *Social Science & Medicine, 259*, 112818.

Lilienfeld, S. O., Basterfield, C., Bowes, S. M., & Costello, T. H. (2020). Nobelists gone wild: Case studies in the domain specificity of critical thinking. In R. J. Sternberg & D. F. Halpern (Eds.), *Critical thinking in psychology* (pp. 10–38). Cambridge University Press.

Marsh, T., Marsh, D. C., Ozawagosh, J., & Ozawagosh, F. (2018). The sweat lodge ceremony: A healing intervention for intergenerational trauma and substance use. *International Indigenous Policy Journal, 9*(2).

McClelland, C. (2021). *Life coaching takes deadly turn after young executive dies following $14,000-course that amplifies negative emotions.* Financial Post. https://financialpost.com/fp-work/life-coaching-takes-deadly-turn-after-young-executive-dies-following-14000-course-that-amplifies-negative-emotions

McDermott-Murphy, C. (2021). Negotiating the irrational with Daniel Kahneman. *Harvard Gazette.* Retrieved from https://news.harvard.edu/gazette/story/2021/12/daniel-kahneman-on-how-to-influence-others/

Meehl, P. (1973). Why I do not attend case conferences. In P. E. Meehl (Ed.), *Psychodiagnosis, selected papers* (pp. 225–302). University of Minnesota Press.

Mosleh, M., Pennycook, G., Arechar, A. A., & Rand, D. (2021). Cognitive reflection correlates with behavior on Twitter. *Nature Communications, 12*, 921.

Nurse, P. (2013). *Attention, Nobel Prize winners! Advice from someone who's already won.* https://www.independent.co.uk/voices/comment/attention-nobel-prize-winners-advice-from-someone-who-s-already-won-8874646.html

Oliver, J. E., & Wood, T. (2014). Medical conspiracy theories and health behaviors in the United States. *JAMA Internal Medicine, 174*, 817–818.

Pennycook, G., Cheyne, J. A., Barr, N., Koehler, D. J., & Fugelsang, J. A. (2015). On the reception and detection of pseudo-profound bullshit. *Judgment and Decision Making, 10*, 549–563.

Pierre, J. M. (2020). Mistrust and misinformation: A two-component, socio-epistemic model of belief in conspiracy theories. *Journal of Social and Political Psychology, 8*.

Ray, J. A. (2020). *The business of redemption: The price of leadership in both life and business.* Morgan James Publishing.

Scherer, L. D., McPhetres, J., Pennycook, G., Kempe, A., Allen, L. A., Knoepke, C. E., Tate, C. E., & Matlock, D. D. D. (2021). Who is susceptible to online health misinformation? A test of four psychosocial hypotheses. *Health Psychology, 40*, 274–284.

Scheufele, D. A., & Krause, N. M. (2019). Science audiences, misinformation, and fake news. *Proceedings of the National Academy of Sciences of the United States of America, 116*(16), 7662–7669.

Semeniuk, I. (2016). Waterloo study on BS wins Ig Nobel Peace Prize. *Globe and Mail.* https://www.theglobeandmail.com/news/national/university-of-waterloo-team-wins-big-for-bs-at-cheeky-ig-nobel-prize-ceremony/article32037498/

Stollznow, K. (2011). Braco the gazer. *Skeptical Inquirer.* https://skepticalinquirer.org/exclusive/braco-the-gazer/

Stroud, M. (2013). *The death dealer.* The Verge. https://www.theverge.com/2013/12/4/5038930/the-death-dealer-james-arthur-sweat-lodge-deaths-in-sedona

Tozer, T. (2023). Artist, 32, took her own life after drinking hallucinogenic "tea" in trendy shamanic healing ritual at £620-a-head retreat, inquest hears. *Daily Mail.* https://www.dailymail.co.uk/news/article-11607545/Artist-took-life-drinking-hallucinogenic-tea-shamanic-healing-ritual-inquest-hears.html

Vosoughi, S., Roy, D., & Aral, S. (2018). The spread of true and false news online. *Science, 359*, 1146–1151.

Walker, A. C., Turpin, M. H., Stolz, J. A., Fugelsang, J. A., & Koehler, D. J. (2019). Finding meaning in the clouds: Illusory pattern perception predicts receptivity to pseudo-profound bullshit. *Judgment and Decision Making, 14*, 109–119.

Zhou, C., Jiang, T., & Zhu, L. (2018). Direct Gaze blurs self-other boundaries. *Journal of General Psychology, 145*, 280–295.

Chapter 7

Akhtar, A. (2022). *Ayurvedic medicine is taking the wellness industry by storm. Here's what you need to know about the traditional Indian practice.* https://www.insider.com/what-is-ayurvedic-medicine-doctors-explain-the-indian-practice-2022-3

Andrade, G. (2017). Is past life regression therapy ethical? *Journal of Medical Ethics and History of Medicine, 10*, 11.

Anestis, M. D., Anestis, J. C., Zawilinski, L. L., Hopkins, T., & Lilienfeld, S. O. (2014). Equine-related treatments for mental disorders lack empirical support: A systematic review of empirical investigations. *Journal of Clinical Psychology, 70*, 1115–1132.

Bergman, B., G., Fallah-Sohy, N., Hoffman, L. A., & Kelly, J. F. (2019). Psychosocial approaches in the treatment of opioid use disorders. In J. F. Kelly & S. Wakeman (Eds.), *Treating opioid addiction* (pp. 109–138). Springer Nature.

Brent, J. (2013). Commentary on the abuse of metal chelation therapy in patients with autism spectrum disorders. *Journal of Medical Toxicology, 9*, 370–372.

Canadian Association of Naturopathic Doctors. (n.d.). *About naturopathic medicine.* https://www.cand.ca/about-naturopathic-medicine/

Dieudonne, M. (2020). Electromagnetic hypersensitivity: A critical review of explanatory hypotheses. *Environmental Health, 19.*

Editorial. (2019). The World Health Organization's decision about traditional Chinese medicine could backfire. *Nature, 570*(7759), 5.

Endocrine Society. (2022). *Adrenal fatigue*. https://www.endocrine.org/patient-engagement/endocrine-library/adrenal-fatigue

Ernst, E. (2008). Chiropractic: A critical evaluation. *Journal of Pain and Symptom Management, 35*, 544–562.

Farias, M., Maraldi, E., Wallenkampf, K. C., & Lucchetti, G. (2020). Adverse events in meditation practices and meditation-based therapies: A systematic review. *Acta Psychiatrica Scandinavica, 142*, 374–393.

Feder, H. M. Jr., Johnson, B. J., O'Connell, S., Shapiro, E. D., Steere, A. C., Wormser, G. P., Ad Hoc International Lyme Disease Group, Agger, W. A., Artsob, H., Auwaerter, P., Dumler, J. S., Bakken, J. S., Bockenstedt, L. K., Green, J., Dattwyler, R. J., Muonz, J., Nadelman, R. B., Schwartz, I., Draper, T., . . . Zeml, L.(2007). A critical appraisal of "chronic Lyme disease." *New England Journal of Medicine, 357*, 1422–1430.

First, M. B., Drevets, W. C., Carter, C., Dickstein, D. P., Kasoff, L., McConathy, J., Rauch, S., Saad, Z. S., Savitz, J., Seymour, K. E., Sheline, Y. I., & Zubieta, J. K. (2018). Clinical applications of neuroimaging in psychiatric disorders. *American Journal of Psychiatry, 175*, 915–916.

Garrett, B., & Riou, M. (2021). A rapid evidence assessment of recent therapeutic touch research. *Nursing Open, 8*, 2318–2330.

Goldberg, S. B., Pace, B. T., Nicholas, C. R., Raison, C. L., & Hutson, P. R. (2020). The experimental effects of psilocybin on symptoms of anxiety and depression: A meta-analysis. *Psychiatry Research, 284*, 112749.

Goodwin, G. M., Aaronson, S. T., Alvarez, O., Arden, P. C., Baker, A., Bennett, J. C., Bird, C., Blom, R. E., Brennan, C., Brusch, D., Burke, L., Campbell-Coker, K., Carhart-Harris, R., Cattell, J., Daniel, A., DeBattista, C., Dunlp, B. W., Eisen, K., Feifel, D., . . . Malievskaia, E. (2022). Single-dose psilocybin for a treatment-resistant episode of major depression. *New England Journal of Medicine, 387*, 1637–1648.

Gorski, D. (2018). *Functional medicine: Reams of useless tests in one hand, a huge invoice in the other*. Science-Based Medicine. https://sciencebasedmedicine.org/functional-medicine-reams-of-useless-tests-in-one-hand-a-huge-invoice-in-the-other/

Guadiano, B. A., & Herbert, J. D. (2000). Can we really tap our problems away? A critical analysis of thought field therapy. *Skeptical Inquirer, 24*. Retrieved from https://skepticalinquirer.org/2000/07/can-we-really-tap-our-problems-away/

Hall, H. (2018). *Leaky brain, leaky gut: Are they real?* Science-Based Medicine. https://sciencebasedmedicine.org/leaky-brain-leaky-gut-are-they-real/

Health Canada. (2019). *Hyperbaric oxygen therapy*. https://www.canada.ca/en/health-canada/services/healthy-living/your-health/medical-information/hyperbaric-oxygen-therapy.html

Hoogeveen, S., Haaf, J. M., Bulbulia, J. A., Ross, R. M., McKay, R., Altay, S., Bendixen, T., Berniunas, R., Cheshin, A., Gentili, C., Georgescu, R., Gervais, W. M., Hagel, K., Kavanagh, C., Levy, N., Neely, A., Qiu, L., Rabelo, A., Ramsay, J. E., . . . van Elk, M. (2022). The Einstein effect provides global evidence for scientific source credibility effects and the influence of religiosity. *Nature Human Behavior, 6*, 523–535.

Lilienfeld, S. O. (2011). Distinguishing scientific from pseudoscientific psychotherapies: Evaluating the role of theoretical plausibility, with a little help from Reverend Bayes. *Clinical Psychology: Science and Practice, 18*, 105–112.

Lilienfeld, S. O., Marshall, J., Todd, J. T., & Shane, H. C. (2014). The persistence of fad interventions in the face of negative scientific evidence: Facilitated communication for autism as a case example. *Evidence-Based Communication Assessment and Intervention, 8*, 62–101.

Liu, Q., Lawrence, A. J., & Liang, J. H. (2011). Traditional Chinese medicine for treatment of alcoholism: From ancient to modern. *American Journal of Chinese Medicine, 39*, 1–13.

Lynn, S. J., Ashwin, G., Ellenberg, S., & Lilienfeld, S. O. (2018). Hypnosis: Science, pseudoscience, and nonsense. In A. B. Kaufman & J. C. Kaufman (Eds.), *Pseudoscience: The conspiracy against science* (pp. 331–349). Boston Review.

Marcon, A. R., Murdoch, B., & Caulfield, T.(2019). The "subluxation" issue: An analysis of chiropractic clinic websites. *Archives of Physiotherapy, 9*, 11.

Marino, L., & Lilienfeld, S. O. (2021). Third time's the charm or three strikes you're out? An updated review of the efficacy of dolphin-assisted therapy for autism and developmental disabilities. *Journal of Clinical Psychology, 77*, 1265–1279.

McGeown, W. J., Mazzoni, G., Venneri, A., & Kirsch, I. (2009). Hypnotic induction decreases anterior default mode activity. *Consciousness and Cognition, 18*, 848–855.

Meichenbaum, D., & Lilienfeld, S. O. (2018). How to spot hype in the field of psychotherapy: A 19-item checklist. *Professional Psychology: Research and Practice, 49*(1), 22–30.

Miller, L. (2010). Remembrances of lives past. *New York Times.* https://www.nytimes.com/2010/08/29/fashion/29PastLives.html

Morton, E., Sakai, K., Ashtari, A., Pleet, M., Michalak, E. E., & Woolley, J. (2023). Risks and benefits of psilocybin use in people with bipolar disorder: An international web-based survey on experiences of "magic mushroom" consumption. *Journal of Psychopharmacology, 37*, 49–60.

Muldowney, D. (2023). *Brain doctor to the stars labeled a "snake-oil" salesman.* Daily Beast. https://www.thedailybeast.com/dr-daniel-amen-called-a-snake-oil-salesman-by-critics-and-former-patients-over-spect-brain-scans

National Center for Complementary and Integrative Health. (2019). *Tradition Chinese medicine: What you need to know.* https://www.nccih.nih.gov/health/traditional-chinese-medicine-what-you-need-to-know

National Center for Complementary and Integrative Health. (2023). *Ayurvedic medicine: In depth.* https://www.nccih.nih.gov/health/ayurvedic-medicine-in-depth

Norcross, J. C., et al. (2006). Discredited psychological treatments and tests: A Delphi poll. *Professional Psychology: Research and Practice, 37*, 515.

Novella, S. (2010). *Plausibility in science-based medicine.* Science-Based Medicine. https://sciencebasedmedicine.org/plausibility-in-science-based-medicine/

Oakley, D. A., & Halligan, P. W. (2013). Hypnotic suggestion: Opportunities for cognitive neuroscience. *Nature Reviews Neuroscience, 14*, 565–576.

Otgaar, H., Howe, M. L., & Patihis, L. (2022). What science tells us about false and repressed memories. *Memory, 30*, 16–21.

Pew Research Center. (2021). *Views on the afterlife.* https://www.pewresearch.org/religion/2021/11/23/views-on-the-afterlife/

Przeworski, A., Peterson, E., & Piedra, A. (2021). A systematic review of the efficacy, harmful effects, and ethical issues related to sexual orientation change efforts. *Clinical Psychology: Science and Practice, 28*, 81–100.

Rosa, L., Rosa, E., Sarner, L., & Barrett, S. (1998). A close look at therapeutic touch. *JAMA, 279*, 1005–1010.

Rosen, G. M., & Davison, G. C. (2003). Psychology should list empirically supported principles of change (ESPs) and not credential trademarked therapies or other treatment packages. *Behavior Modification, 27*(3), 300–312.

Rosenfeld, E. A., & McLean, C. (2024). Purple hat therapies. In J. N. Stea & S. Hupp (Eds.), *Investigating clinical psychology: Pseudoscience, fringe science, and controversies*. Routledge.

The Guardian. (2019). *Berlin Wall pills: A cure for emotional trauma—or royal-endorsed quackery*. https://www.theguardian.com/lifeandstyle/shortcuts/2019/aug/21/berlin-wall-pills

U.S. Food and Drug Administration. (2023). *Code of federal regulations, Title 21*. https://www.accessdata.fda.gov/scripts/cdrh/cfdocs/cfcfr/cfrsearch.cfm?fr=801.415

Van Dam, N. T., van Vugt, M. K., Vago, D. R., Schmalzl, L., Saron, C. D., Olendzki, A., Meissner, T., Lazar, S. W., Kerr, C. E., Gorchov, J., Fox, C. R., Field, B. A., Britton, W. B., Brefczynski-Lewis, J. A., & Meyer, D. E. (2018). Mind the hype: A critical evaluation and prescriptive agenda for research on mindfulness and meditation. *Perspectives on Psychological Science, 13*, 36–61.

Weiss, B. L. (1992). *Through time into healing: Discovering the power of regression therapy to erase trauma and transform mind, body, and relationships*. Touchstone.

Witkowski, T. (2010). Thirty-five years of research on neuro-linguistic programming. NLP research database. State of the art or pseudoscientific decoration. *Polish Psychological Bulletin, 41*, 58–66.

Wood, J. M., Nezworski, T., Lilienfeld, S. O., & Garb, H. N. (2003). *What's wrong with the Rorschach? Science confronts the controversial inkblot test*. Jossey-Bass.

Chapter 8

Beck, A. T. (2019). A 60-year evolution of cognitive theory and therapy. *Perspectives on Psychological Science, 14*, 16–20.

Berezow, A. B. (2012). Why psychology isn't a science. *Los Angeles Times*. https://www.latimes.com/opinion/la-xpm-2012-jul-13-la-ol-blowback-pscyhology-science-20120713-story.html

Bower, P., & Gilbody, S. (2018). Stepped care in psychological therapies: Access, effectiveness, and efficiency: Narrative literature review. *British Journal of Psychiatry, 186*, 11–17.

Cuijpers, P., Miguel, C., Harrer, M., Plessen, C. Y., Ciharova, M., Ebert, D., & Karyotaki, E. (2023). Cognitive behavior therapy vs. control conditions, other psychotherapies, pharmacotherapies and combined treatment for depression: A comprehensive meta-analysis including 409 trials with 52,702 patients. *World Psychiatry, 22*, 105–115.

Edinger, J. D., Arnedt, J. T., Bertisch, S. M., Carney, C. E., Harrington, J. J., Lichstein, K. L., Sateia, M. J., Troxel, W. M., Zhou, E. S., Kazmi, U., Heald, J. L., & Martin, J. L. (2021). Behavioral and psychological treatments for chronic insomnia disorder in adults: An American Academy of Sleep Medicine systematic review, meta-analysis, and GRADE assessment. *Journal of Clinical Sleep Medicine, 17*, 263–298.

Eubanks, C. F., & Goldfried, M. (2019). A principle-based approach to psychotherapy integration. In J. C. Norcross & M. Goldfried (Eds.), *Handbook of psychotherapy integration* (3rd ed., pp. 88–104). Oxford University Press.

Hare-Duke, L., Dening, T., de Oliveira, D., Milner, K., & Slade, M. (2019). Conceptual framework for social connectedness in mental disorders: Systematic review and narrative synthesis. *Journal of Affective Disorders, 245,* 188–199.

Jones, J. L., & Mehr, S. L. (2007). Foundations and assumptions of the scientist-practitioner model. *American Behavioral Scientist, 50,* 766–771.

Lilienfeld, S. O. (2010). Can psychology become a science? *Personality and Individual Differences, 49,* 281–288.

Lilienfeld, S. O. (2011). Public skepticism of psychology. Why many people perceive the study of human behavior as unscientific. *American Psychologist, 67,* 111–129.

Lilienfeld, S. O. (2019). What is "evidence" in psychotherapies? *World Psychiatry, 18,* 245–246.

Magill, M., & Ray, L. A. (2009). Cognitive-behavioral treatment with adult alcohol and illicit drug users: A meta-analysis of randomized controlled trials. *Journal of Studies on Alcohol and Drugs, 70,* 516–527.

Martins, L. B., Braga Tibaes, J. R., Sanches, M., Jacka, F., Berk, M., & Teixeira, A. L. (2021). Nutrition-based interventions for mood disorders. *Expert Review of Neurotherapeutics, 21,* 303–315.

Norcross, J. C., & Karpiak, C. P. (2023). Relationship factors. In S. D. Miller, D. Chow, S. Malins, & M. A. Hubble (Eds.), *The field guide to better results: Evidence-based exercises to improve therapeutic effectiveness* (pp. 107–130). American Psychological Association.

Pead, S., & Hawley, S. (2023). *Survey finds a third of teen boys look up to internet celebrity and self-described misogynist Andrew Tate.* ABC News Daily. https://www.abc.net.au/news/2023-01-25/andrew-tate-admired-by-teenage-boys-survey-shows/101885940

Schuch, F. B., & Vancampfort, D. (2021). Physical activity, exercise, and mental disorders: It is time to move on. *Trends in Psychiatry and Psychotherapy, 43,* 177–184.

Shedler, J. (2010). The efficacy of psychodynamic psychotherapy. *American Psychologist, 65,* 98–109.

Shedler, J. (2022). That was then, this is now: Psychoanalytic psychotherapy for the rest of us. *Contemporary Psychoanalysis, 58,* 405–437.

Society of Clinical Psychology. (2022). *Psychological treatments.* https://div12.org/treatments/

Sung, M. (2022). *The internet can't stop talking about Andrew Tate.* NBC News. https://www.nbcnews.com/pop-culture/viral/internet-cant-stop-talking-andrew-tate-tiktok-rcna42744

Wasil, A. R., Venturo-Conerly, K. E., Shingleton, R. M., & Weisz, J. R. (2019). A review of popular smartphone apps for depression and anxiety: Assessing the inclusion of evidence-based content. *Behaviour Research and Therapy, 123,* 103498.

Wieten, S. (2018). Expertise in evidence-based medicine: A tale of three models. *Philosophy, Ethics, and Humanities in Medicine, 13*(1), 2. https://doi.org/10.1186/s13010-018-0055-2

Williams, A. J., Botanov, Y., Giovanetti, A. K., Perko, V. L., Sutherland, C. L., Youngren, W., & Sakaluk, J. K. (2023). A metascientific review of the evidential value of acceptance and commitment therapy for depression. *Behavior Therapy, 54,* 989–1005.

Youyou, W., Yang, Y., & Uzzi, B. (2023). A discipline-wide investigation of the replicability of psychology papers over the past two decades. *PNAS, 120,* e2208863120. https://doi.org/10.1073/pnas.2208863120

Chapter 9

Forrest, S. (2012). *Yesterday's sky: Astrology and Ireincarnation*. Seven Paws Press.

Giamcomucci, S. (2021). *Psychodrama as an effective treatment for trauma and PTSD experience.* https://www.apadivisions.org/division-49/news-events/psychodrama-trauma-treatment

Orbiki, H., & Feninger-Schaal, R. (2019). Integrative systematic review of psychodrama psychotherapy research: Trends and methodological implications. *PLOS One*, *14*, e0212575.

Tambling, R. R., D'Aniello, C., & Russell, B. S. (2023). Mental health literacy: A critical target for narrowing racial disparities in behavioral health. *International Journal of Mental Health and Addiction*, *21*, 1867–1881.

U.S. Government Accountability Office. (2022). *Mental health care: Access challenges for covered consumers and relevant federal efforts*. https://www.gao.gov/assets/gao-22-104597-highlights.pdf

Turuba, R., Zenone, M., Srivastava, R., Stea, J. N., Quintana, Y., Ow, N., Marchand, K., Kwan, A., Ong, A-J., Ding, X., Warren, C., Marcon, A., Henderson, J. L., Mathias, S., & Barbic, S. (submitted). Do you have depression? A summative content analysis of mental health-related content on TikTok.

Index

For the benefit of digital users, indexed terms that span two pages (e.g., 52–53) may, on occasion, appear on only one of those pages.

Figures are indicated with an italic *f* following the page/paragraph number.